The Home Alternative
—— to ——
Hospitals and Nursing Homes

The Home Alternative

to

Hospitals and Nursing Homes

Mara Covell

Medical Consultants:
Maurice Beer, M.D., and Eileen Hanley, R.N.

An Owl Book

Holt, Rinehart and Winston
NEW YORK

Published by Holt, Rinehart and Winston,
383 Madison Avenue, New York, New York 10017.
Published simultaneously in Canada by Holt,
Rinehart and Winston of Canada, Limited.

Library of Congress Cataloging in Publication Data
Covell, Mara.
The home alternative to hospitals and nursing homes.
Includes index.
1. Home nursing. 2. Home care services. I. Beer,
Maurice. II. Hanley, Eileen. III. Title. [DNLM:
1. Home Nursing. WY 200 C873h]
RT61.C68 1985   649'.8   84-19757
ISBN 0-03-003922-3 (An Owl bk.) (pbk.)

First published in hardcover by Rawson Associates
in 1983.
First Owl Book Edition—1985

Designer: Jacques Chazaud
Printed in the United States of America
10 9 8 7 6 5 4 3 2 1

ISBN 0-03-003922-3

*For my father
with all my love*

Contents

ACKNOWLEDGMENTS   ix

PREFACE   xi

1. What Is Home Care—and Why Is It Here
   to Stay?   1
2. How to Take Charge of Home Care!   6
3. Your Bible for Home-Care Tasks   33
4. Nursing Skills to Turn You into the Doctor's
   Care-Partner   80
5. How to Gain Health-Clue Savvy—and Be a
   Super Care Giver   95
6. How to Help Your Patient Eat for Recovery   126
7. Care-Confidence: Taking Care of Your
   Patient After Surgery   148
8. Home-Care Styles for a Sick Child   166
9. Sexuality and Home Care   202
10. Emergency Medical Care: Life-Saving Steps
    for Your Patient   227
11. How to Care for a Mentally Ill Relative at
    Home   249
12. Loving Home Care for the Older Adult   275

13. Caring for a Loved One Who Has a Terminal
    Illness   309
14. Additional Resources   318

    INDEX   331

ACKNOWLEDGMENTS

One of the joys of having written this book was that I met so many remarkable people. These professionals, who bring a profound dedication to their work, also gave me generous amounts of their time, expertise, and insight. Although it is not possible to name them all, I would like to extend my deepest appreciation to the following.

To the physicians: Howard Kesseler, John Eden, Willibald Nagler, and Elizabeth Watkins; to the nurses: Louise Kruger, Diana Brown, Maura McCormack, Virginia Hart Clark, Marilyn Liota, Missilene Edwards, Mary Ellen Wadsworth, Sister Patrice O'Connor, Jane Morris, Sally Bishop; the social workers: Pamela Boyle, Marjorie Jonas, Purnima Chopra, Susan Blumenfield, Jill Elliot; the therapists: Rochelle Bukatman, Christine Khaleeli; the registered dietician: Susan Roger Rooney; the certified sexuality counselor: Pamela Boyle.

I would also like to thank my medical consultants, Maurice Beer and Eileen Hanley, for their dedication to this project; staff members at the Sophie Palmer Library in New York City, Cosy Brown and Debbie Kurtz, whose kindness and support made my many hours of library research a joy; Marie-Claire Margules, who generously contributed office space and friendship; my agent and editor, Alyss Dorese and Eleanor Rawson, respectively, whose faith in me and belief in home care helped turn this book into a reality; Jackie Aher, who contributed the illustrations that grace these pages; and a special thank you to my family, whose love and affection are an ever present source of strength and inspiration.

Preface

What is an alternative to hospitals and nursing homes? The answer is clear: home care.

When serious illness threatened my father's well-being, my family and I discovered the comfort, dignity, and humaneness that only home care could provide. We also found that home care was dramatically less expensive than hospital care. And, today, with skyrocketing medical costs and health-service cutbacks, that was a blessing.

While caring for my father, I lived through the many questions, frustrations, and concerns, with the questions they give rise to, that so often accompany home care: how to administer medication, utilize community services—in short, how to cope. There were times of intense emotional and physical stress. Professionals were not always available or approachable for advice.

Instinctively, I searched for a book to guide me, a book to give me emotional support and practical information. But such a book was hard to find. That is why I've written this one. It springs from my personal experiences and my belief in home care's profound rewards.

Because my family and I chose home care instead of hospital care we were able to give my father the loving and individualized treatment that he wouldn't have received in an institutional setting. Our rewards were the joy of his recovery and the emotional closeness we all felt as a result of our care-giving adventure.

If this book gives you the incentive to consider home care as an alternative to hospitals and nursing homes in appropriate situations, then it will have served its purpose.

If it provides you with confidence and support during your home-care experience, I will be rewarded once more.

Mara Brand Covell

1

What Is Home Care— and Why Is It Here to Stay?

Not long ago my father was seriously ill. My family and I knew that a long hospital stay would deplete our savings, that recovery among strangers would only add to Dad's trauma. So we opted for home care. It seemed the least expensive alternative—and the most loving.

Under the supervision of a physician, my family and I united to meet Dad's special health needs. It wasn't always easy. Lots of medication and treatment had to be given according to strict instructions. We kept night and day vigils to ward off crises.

There were weeks of worrying, of seeing Dad in pain and of experiencing feelings of love so profound that to this day I am awed by them.

Eventually, through our support and his own iron will, Dad recovered.

Never have I regretted keeping my father at home instead of in the hospital. Indeed, the benefits of home care have lasted beyond his recovery: The joy of contributing to his well-being and the outpouring of love shared within the family made the home-care experience one of the most remarkable of my life.

Home care is a health-style alternative that adapts to simple illnesses as well as complicated, prolonged ones. Home care can fit into your life. Read on to see how.

What Exactly Is Home Care?

Home care allows many people to stay at home during the course of their illnesses. Most often, this is made possible by a physician who supervises family members willing to provide patient care and by home health agencies, which offer specialized services. Consequently, home care permits patients to remain home while continuing a life-style as close to normal as possible.

Why Not Hospital Care?

The hospital scene is just that—a scene. Personhood disappears the moment a patient dons a hospital gown. Dignity flies out the window at the first icy touch of a bedpan. Peace, quiet, and privacy? Forget it. And the loneliness—the penetrating loneliness. Patients must truly depend on the kindness of strangers.

Not to be flippant. Hospitals save lives. They are an important part of our health-care system. Indeed, they offer constant medical supervision by highly skilled professionals, diagnostic tools, and sophisticated facilities for the critically ill. The trouble is the quality of hospital life. And the astronomical cost. Bad news on both counts.

Enter home care. It's a health style that has been emerging slowly for years. It is finally taking hold in the eighties because it meets today's special needs.

How Does Home Care Meet the Special Needs of the Eighties?

Frankly, I'm talking about financial needs. Health services in this country have not been spared President Reagan's budget cutting ax. If you think that only the elderly and the poor have been hardest hit, think again. We've all been affected—and we'll continue to be. Spending for health care in 1981 in this country was up 15.1% from the previous year. The most notable thing about health care spending has been its rapid and sustained rate of growth. The bottom line: We are faced with a decrease in health services—and an increase in medical costs.

Home care is an alternative that can help you cope with these grim economic realities. It's dramatically less expensive than hospital and institutional care. For example, the average hospital cost per day is $350 compared to $40 to care for a loved one in the home setting.

Do You Know These Home-Care Benefits?

FACT: Home care is less expensive than hospital and institutional care.

FACT: Home care can enhance the healing process and lead to a speedier recovery.

FACT: Home care reduces the length of hospital stays—and in some cases makes them unnecessary.

FACT: Home care gives us stronger control over our bodies because it promotes dignity, self-care, and individuality.

FACT: Home care is appropriate when a hospital is not close by or when hospital beds are not readily available.

FACT: Home care is more conducive to patient education than hospital care. The patient at home is more receptive to learning ways to improve poor health habits and prevent recurrence of illness.

When Is Home Care the Right Choice?

Certainly, home care is not for everyone. After all, home is as much a state of mind as a place. And it may be preferable for some people to be hospitalized rather than convalesce amidst family tensions, personality conflicts, or poor conditions.

Even more important, people who are seriously ill and require round-the-clock medical supervision should be hospitalized, to be where the latest medical equipment and trained health-care personnel are always available.

So when is home care the right choice? When it's a choice made in collaboration with a physician which ensures that:
• intricate services of the hospital are *not* needed
• home can comfortably sustain or improve the patient's health
• the patient's family or friends will provide necessary care
• the patient has access to the local in-home health services he or she needs.

What Kinds of People Turn to Home Care?

All kinds. All ages. From all walks of life. In fact, 90% of physicians surveyed believe that home care can satisfactorily meet the needs of most of their patients. These may be:
• patients recovering from accidents, injuries
• patients recovering from surgery
• patients recovering from mental disorders
• patients with chronic diseases
• patients being treated for cancer
• new mothers and their babies home from the hospital
• patients who are newly disabled
• patients with severe arthritis
• patients who have had strokes
• patients recovering from heart attacks and other cardiac disorders
• patients needing home dialysis for kidney disease
• patients receiving chemotherapy or radiation therapy
• patients receiving immunotherapy
• patients who have received out-patient hospital services
• patients who need rehabilitation to relearn old skills (walking, talking, performing household tasks, etc.)
• patients who need a change in diet or nutrition to prevent worsening or recurring illness

- patients with terminal illnesses
- patients coping with the deteriorating illnesses of aging
- patients recovering from simple illnesses such as colds and flu.

2

How to Take Charge of Home Care!

I am concerned about the number of people in need of home care who find themselves asking, "What do I do now? Where do I turn for help?" Why so much ignorance? Because hospitals too often discontinue their responsibilities with the patient's discharge. And too few physicians have the time to develop home-care programs for their patients.

During my home-care experience I dealt with a physician who supervised medical treatment, but who did little to point me in the direction of local support services. He told me to hire a nurse, but he didn't tell me how, what criteria to use, or where to go. He told me to perform a variety of care tasks, but he never prepared me for their emotional or physical repercussions. I mention him because he is more typical than not and he was a kindly person. Chances are he's not unlike the physician with whom you will deal or may be dealing.

There is only one solution to the problem of inadequate support and information from medical professionals: knowledge. You must know what services are available so that you can gain control of your home-care situation. That's what this chapter is all about. It offers the basic information you will need to get a home-care program started in the most humane, speediest, and efficient way.

Let me begin by saying there are three ways to get home care going—the hospital-, the physician-, or the patient-coordinated program. Each has its pluses and minuses. Here's the lowdown.

The Hospital-Coordinated Program

Hospital care is more than outright medical service. It is also discharge planning. Every hospital has a discharge plan for each patient. The type of plan varies from institution to institution but the goal is always the same: assess the patient's case and decide whether or not home care will be needed.

Who makes this decision? Most often a team of medical professionals that includes your patient's physician, nurse(s), and the hospital social worker. They review the case. They decide if the patient will need special care at home. If he or she does, the team will determine if such care is feasible. In other words, does the patient want it, can the patient afford it, are there local health services available, and can someone provide care at home?

Let me add that although the hospital team may decide your patient needs home care, they may do very little to get such a program going. On the other hand, some hospitals may pitch in to help you locate resources and health-service providers, arrange care, receive financial advice, and even stay in touch with you until your patient's recovery is complete. I suggest that you find out which type of hospital programs are available in your area. How? Consult the physician or local hospital's discharge planning department. Also, some hospitals have a "Home-Care Department." Try that, too.

The Physician-Coordinated Program

Not all candidates for home care have been previously hospitalized. In fact, many kinds of chronic conditions, injuries, disabilities, mental illnesses, and infectious diseases can be managed at home without prior hospitalization.

Physician-coordinated home care simply means that the doctor believes there is a need for care at home. He or she has consulted with the patient and/or family to determine if it is feasible. Once the go-ahead is given the physician may make referrals to local home-health agencies (i.e., The Visiting Nurse Service), skilled health services (i.e., physical therapists), adult day-care centers, and so on.

The physician's involvement in home care depends on the patient's condition and the doctor's own style of care-giving. Some doctors get more involved than others. Yours may make referrals and occasional visits, or may just supervise—thereby leaving all the coordinating and legwork up to you.

I urge you to select a home-care physician who is accessible and willing to give you the time and support your patient needs for proper home care. How do you find such a person? See the suggestions that follow.

What to Do When YOU Must Coordinate Home Care: A Five-Step Plan

I know that this seems like an awesome responsibility. Don't panic. There are many agencies and organizations to help you manage.

I coordinated home care. You can, too. Here's my Five-Step Plan:

1. *Always* have a physician ready to supervise the medical aspects of care.

2. Plug into the available home-care services by contacting a social worker, discharge planning or home-care department at the local hospital, the county social services department, or the local public health department.

3. Delegate home-care responsibilities to other family members, friends, or neighbors whenever possible.

4. Know your patient's financial resources and explore additional sources of financial reimbursement and support. (See the end of this chapter for more information.)

5. You may need support to help with the emotional repercussions of care. There are many self-help groups to enable you to do just that. To locate the ones best suited to your needs consult a physician, nurse, or the public relations department at your

local hospital, and/or your community mental health center. For a listing of self-help groups intended to benefit people with minor problems as well as overwhelming tragedies, write for *Help: A Working Guide to Self-Help Groups*, by Alan Gartner and Frank Riessman, % New Viewpoints, Dept. E–J, 730 Fifth Ave., New York, N.Y. 10019 ($9.95). Another excellent source is the National Self-Help Clearinghouse, which can help you locate a support group that meets your special needs. The address: National Self-Help Clearinghouse, Graduate School and University Center of the City University of New York, 33 West 42nd St., Rm. 1227, New York, N.Y. 10036; Telephone: (212) 840–7606.

The Home-Care Team

There are always at least two team members: the *patient* and the *physician*. When needed, this partnership opens to include a close family member or friend called the *care giver*.

What if the services of in-home professionals are needed? Then you may hire the following helpers: *visiting nurses, home-health aides, speech/physical/occupational/respiratory therapists, registered dieticians* or *social workers*. For custodial care you may turn to *paid home attendants* (companions), *housekeepers*, or *volunteers*.

The formula for quality home care is the efficient coordination of highly skilled team members. To guarantee delivery you need to know each member's job and how to hire the best ones. Want to know more? Read on.

The Patient

To be ill is to encounter life's deepest vulnerability. Illness can bring pain, fear, depression, and dependency. Few things seem as important as the need to be well.

Despite this, your patient must work harder than any other team member to improve and maintain health. My father, for example, mustered all his strength, followed doctor's orders, adhered to his medication schedule and new diet—and overcame his illness. I look back on that miracle and realize that it wasn't as much an act of God as it was my father's need to assume control and responsibility for himself whenever humanly possible. He was a good patient who beat the odds.

Certainly, every illness does not have a happy ending. But I am convinced that the best patients manage their illnesses and try not to let their illnesses manage them.

Encourage your loved one to be a good patient by prompting him or her to:

• be as independent as possible. Participate in as many activities as the illness and physician allow; try to perform simple tasks such as bathing, dressing, shaving, shampooing, and light housekeeping. Movement helps maintain flexibility and mobility that often diminish during home confinement.

• act sensibly during illness. Follow prescribed treatments and medications. However, postpone any treatment that seems inappropriate or causes side-effects until you can discuss it in detail with the physician or get another opinion.

• explain disturbing symptoms and emotions to the physician and care giver—within reason.

• try to understand the care giver's feelings. A sensitive care giver may endure intense emotional and physical stress during home care. Accept care graciously. Avoid excessive demands. And always allow the care giver time to rest.

The Physician

The physician will devise a treatment plan and periodically review it with you.

I strongly suggest that you find one who is receptive to and experienced in home care. To make that job easier, here is a checklist.

The Foolproof Way to Find
the Right Home-Care Physician

Physicians are not officially certified as home-care qualified. However, some are better suited to home care than others. Who are they?

• Home-care qualified physicians are primary care doctors. They are licensed internists, general or family practitioners. Why? Because primary care doctors have broad medical care experiences and, generally, more exposure to the problems of home care. Yes, there are specialists (gynecologists, neurologists, surgeons, etc.) who can provide sound medical advice and support. But your best bet is the primary care physician.

• Home-care qualified physicians are easily available. They must be receptive to occasional home visits, if necessary. And they should be willing to supply their phone numbers in case of emergency.

• Home-care qualified physicians are emotionally accessible. They are sincerely concerned about their patients. They are communicative, objective, and compassionate—not an easy order to fill. And not all physicians are able to fill it. To find this type of doctor consult other medical professionals—physicians and nurses. These people are plugged into the medical network of their communities and have firsthand information about physicians, their qualifications and personalities.

• Home-care qualified physicians are willing to deal with nonmedical problems. Conflicts and problems can arise at home that have little to do with medical treatment. Personality clashes between patient and care giver, inefficient custodial care or housekeeping, and poor living conditions can conspire to undermine your patient's health. The physician must recognize these problems and correct them whenever possible.

The Social Worker

Social workers are trained professionals who can describe community services, refer you and your patient to health professionals and offer information about available funding to help you through a financial crisis. In addition, some are qualified to provide psychological counseling.

Don't underestimate the help social workers can supply. They can be an excellent source of information and support during a difficult time.

Find one by calling your nearest hospital social service department or the local public health department; consult the Visiting Nurse Service or county social service agency. Also, check the Yellow Pages in your telephone book under "Social Services" or "Social Worker."

The Nurse

The most visible nurses in home care are the registered nurse (R.N.) and the licensed practical nurse or vocational nurse (L.P.N. or L.V.N.)

The R.N. completes at least two years of academic training and must be licensed by the state to practice. The nurse visits the home to give treatments ordered by your patient's physician (injections, cardiac management, etc.), answers questions about diet, teaches the patient/family how to handle care tasks between visits, and helps plan for self-care.

The L.P.N. or L.V.N. functions only under the supervision of a registered nurse. This person is licensed by the state after one year of specialized training and provides nursing to patients who do not need the attention of an R.N.

To hire a nurse, consult your physician. He or she may offer valuable referrals. During my home-care experience I was forced to locate a nurse on my own. At first the process intimidated me. Then I learned what to do.

Check the Yellow Pages under "Nurses." You will find a variety of private and non-profit organizations. Generally, these agencies screen their applicants and offer nurses with the skills your patient needs. Many professional nursing agencies claim that their staffers belong to state and national nursing associations. They promise that their nurses have top credentials, and receive a yearly physical examination to guarantee that the nurses are in fine health. Many agencies offer twenty-four-hour telephone service.

I'm sure you want the best for your patient. Therefore, I recommend that you ask the physician, social worker, hospital nurse, or home-care experienced friend to refer you to a quality service similar to those I described.

An excellent source for home nurses is the Visiting Nurse Association, a nonprofit service with branches all over the country. The V.N.A. often has a twenty-four-hour telephone line in case of emergency. The V.N.A. functions only on doctor's orders, so be sure that your physician cooperates. If your patient has difficulty paying for nursing care, some V.N.A. chapters have sliding scale fees. Or contact your local department of social services. Your patient may be eligible for public health department nursing visits.

An example of a reputable private nursing service is Upjohn Healthcare Services. They have more than 250 offices around the country. To find the office nearest you, write Upjohn Health Care Services, Trestlewood Office Park, 5080 Lover's Lane, Kalamazoo, Mich. 49002; or check your phonebook.

One last tip about hiring nurses: Screen the nurse yourself to be sure he or she will supply quality care and is compatible with your patient's emotional needs. For example, during my home-care research I met a woman who was caring for her father, a recent stroke victim. She needed a nurse, and after some consideration decided that her father would be more comfortable with a male nurse. Gender may be important to your patient, just as a gentle personality may be more suitable than an assertive one. A good fit between patient and nurse can make all the difference! So, screen carefully.

The Homemaker-Home Health Aide

This individual works under the supervision of a nurse, social worker, or other health professional. He or she can help your patient perform tasks that have become difficult because of illness or disability, such as personal care (shaving, toileting, bathing, etc.) shopping, light housekeeping, and personal laundry. Aides are trained to be more than housekeepers. Some have received specialized training to work specifically with certain types of patients such as the elderly or disabled. Health aides are specifically trained for patient care and may assist in areas such as administering medication.

Consider a homemaker-home health aide when family, friends—and you—are unavailable to help your patient. Aides may also be hired when your loved one needs an escort to and from appointments.

One word of warning: Aides are not licensed, and in some areas they receive little or no professional supervision. Your safest bet is to ask your physician, hospital, or Visiting Nurse Service for referrals. Also, contact the National HomeCaring Council (see Chapter Fourteen). They offer publications and information to help you select the best-qualified aides.

The Therapists

Your physician or nurse will decide whether or not your patient needs the services of a therapist to relearn or improve skills lost through illness or injury. Ask the physician or contact your local hospital for referrals. Among therapists you may need are the following:

• speech therapist: This professional helps patients correct language problems.

• physical therapist: This individual helps patients regain lost abilities in body functioning.

• nutritional therapist or dietician: This type of therapist teaches patients and care givers how to prepare restricted diets and to adapt prescribed diets to the patient's life-style and personal tastes.

• occupational therapist: The occupational therapist fits patients to assistive devices such as wheelchairs and helps them relearn personal care, homemaking skills, and how to function in daily living activities.

• respiratory therapist: This person assists patients with respiratory and other breathing disorders and instructs them in the use of special equipment and breathing exercises.

The Best Ways to Make Patient Care Fit into Your Schedule

Do you have to add patient care to your other responsibilities? That's not always easy. Yet there are ways to revise your schedule to allow time to care for your loved one.

If you have a job, consider:
• temporarily going from full-time to part-time work
• asking your employer if you can use sick days or vacation days to provide care
• asking family, friends, or neighbors for help
• rearranging work hours
• investigating the possibility of working from home
• contacting county social services or social worker for advice about hiring professionals or volunteers for help
• job sharing. There are a number of people who, for various reasons, are not interested in full-time work. So they share their job with another individual who has similar abilities. To learn how you can restructure full-time jobs and present the idea to an employer, write: New Ways to Work, 149 Ninth St., San Francisco, Calif. 94103.

If you have other family obligations such as children, consider:
• hiring housekeepers or volunteers (often offered by church groups or synagogues) to help with chores
• asking other family members, friends, or neighbors to pitch in
• contacting county social services or social worker for advice.

All Home Care and No Play—A Dangerous Duo

It should come as little surprise to you that caring for a loved one who has a long-term illness can deplete you emotionally and physically. I'm not pooh-poohing home care's benefits—just pointing up the realities.

Recent research says that adequate relief is essential for care givers to prevent "care-giver fatigue." The hazardous scenario runs like this: As you *add* home care to your previous responsibilities you risk becoming as homebound as your patient. If you don't take breaks, get help, or have a change of scene you will start to develop these troublesome emotions: depression, irritability, and resentment. The difficulty is compounded when your patient senses your feelings and, in turn, feels guilty or burdened by them.

I experienced care-giver burnout. It didn't happen overnight. It took days of worry, nights of sleeplessness—and no respite. Within a couple of weeks I felt teary and depressed, and at times I just wanted to scream. Experience and common sense made me realize that I needed to take some time for myself *each day*— and that I needed to get away from the care site at least *once or twice a week*. My advice to you: Be kind to yourself. Distract yourself with an absorbing book, diverting television program, or treat. Get out of the house as often as possible. Go store browsing, take in a movie, go out to eat, meet friends. I guarantee that you will find the change restorative—and essential to maintaining your well-being.

Make Home Care Easier with a Home-Health Chart and Medication Sheet

The Home-Health Chart is the best way to record your patient's progress. It provides an organized, sequential picture of your patient's vital signs, symptoms, and changes. You can refer to it to give specific information to the physician. And you will find that it will help you perform care tasks on time.

I suggest you adapt the Home-Health Chart that follows to fit your patient's own care schedule. Simply take the headings (date, time, temperature, pulse, etc.) that are appropriate for your patient, write them at the top of a sheet of paper, and make boxes to record your readings and comments, as shown in the accompanying model (Figure 1). If you have any questions, speak to the physician or nurse for advice.

Another home-care aide is the Medication Sheet. You can use the sample as a guide (Figure 2). Again, use a separate piece of paper and include the headings as suggested, such as date, medication, and instructions. Each time a drug or treatment is administered, check the appropriate box. At the end of the day be sure the number of checks match the prescribed doses.

How to Turn the Sickroom into a Home-Health Hospital

Naturally, you will want your patient to be very comfortable. Select a sickroom that is quiet and, if possible, away from the street and household noises. Keep in mind that a room with an outside window and a lovely view can do much to perk up flagging spirits.

Sickroom supplies

• bed: In most situations a twin bed will do just fine. Double beds may seem spacious, but they are a pain to maneuver and maintain. The physician may recommend a hospital bed. This is especially suited to long-term patients and patients who need special equipment such as traction devices. They are simple to move, can elevate your patient's head or feet, and are at a height you can easily manage. Rent one from a surgical supply store.

• mattress: Choose a firm one. It will be better suited to periodic turning and wear more evenly. Long-term patients may benefit from special mattresses designed to prevent pressure

Date	Time	Temp- erature	Pulse	Respir- ation	Blood Pressure	Medi- cation	Side Effects to Medi- cation	Nature of Stool (color, odor)	Nature of Urine (color, odor)	Urine Output
april 1	8 A.M.	100.1°F	72	18	130/70	100 mg. Bactrim	none	no move- ment	normal	½ pint
	12 NOON	99° F	—	—	—	100 mg. Bactrim	none	normal	normal	½ pint
	4 P.M.	100°F	72	18	130/70	100 mg. Bactrim 2 aspirin	none	no move- ment	normal	½ pint
	9 P.M.	97°F	72	18	—	100 mg. Bactrim 2 aspirin	none	no move- ment	normal	½ pint
april 2										

sores, such as air, flotation, and foam types. They may be ordered through a surgical supply resource. Ask the physician or nurse for recommendations.

• lighting: Keep the room well lighted. Let the sun in (it has a germicidal effect!). Some patients may be sensitive to light. These include people with glaucoma, measles, meningitis, and vitamin B deficiencies. Also, some drugs may cause photosensitivity on exposure to direct sunlight. Check with physician for guidance.

• furnishings: Provide blankets, bed linens, bedside table with lamp, easy chair, telephone (when appropriate), buzzer, bell, or

Pain & Location	Amount & Quality of Sleep	Vomitus (time & nature)	Sputum nature of	Exercise or Treat-ment	Weight	Emotional or Mental Dis-turbances	Additional Comments
mild pain lower back	6 hrs. fitful	none	coughing yellowish	none	130	none	patient ate half of breakfast
mild, lower back	—	some nausea	none	range of motion 15 min.	—	none	itching at wound
none	1 hr. nap	some nausea	none	none	—	none	changed dressing
none	—	none	none	none	—	—	ate complete dinner

Figure 1. Home-Health Chart

Figure 2. Medication Sheet

Date →	April 1					April 2				
↓ Medication and Instructions	8 am	12 noon	4 pm	9 pm	bed-time	8 am	12 noon	4 pm	9 pm	bed-time
Bactrim, one tablet 4 times daily (take before meals with lots of water)	√	√	√	√						
aspirin two when needed for pain			√	√						

intercom to signal care giver. Soothing and attractive colors are best for walls or linens. They create a restful environment.

• standard home-care supplies: Ask the physician or nurse what you need. These things are useful to have on hand:

absorbent cotton
adhesive tape
alcohol
antiseptic soap
bandages
Band-Aids
bath thermometer
bedpan
body lotion
Chux pads or other moisture-
    resistant pads
cotton swabs
drinking glass
enema bag
facial tissue
gauze pads
heating pad
ice pack

medicine dropper
peroxide
personal-care supplies
    (comb, brush, shaving equip-
    ment, etc.)
safety pins
scissors
sphygmomanometer (for
    blood pressure)
stethoscope
talcum powder
teaspoon
thermometer
tweezers
urinal
vaporizer
Vaseline

• how to elevate an ordinary bed: By adjusting the bed to a height that is comfortable for you, you can diminish fatigue and back strain. Determine correct height by placing your palms flat on the mattress. If your shoulders do not change position, the bed is at a proper height. Hospital beds are easy to adjust. To handle an ordinary one, stack magazines, newspapers, wood, or bricks under the legs until the correct height is reached.

• how to incline bed: You may need to elevate one end of the bed. Ask physician or nurse for specific instructions.

• how to lengthen the bed: What do you do if your patient is so tall that his or her legs dangle over the end? Simply extend the mattress by slipping a board underneath it or placing a chair at the end. Cover the board or chair with pillows to hold the patient's feet.

• how to protect the mattress: You can use a waterproof sheet to protect the mattress from wet treatments, incontinent patients, food spills, and draining wounds. Buy one at the surgical supply—or make your own. Use an old vinyl shower curtain, plastic from the dry cleaner, or similar covering. Pin to top of mattress or sew on using an easy-to-remove basting stitch.

• bed linens: Select calm colors, such as cool green, pale blue, yellow. Use solids or simple patterns. They are more comforting than frenzied designs. Fitted bottom sheets bunch less and wrinkle less. Try flannel or satin sheets for a treat or variety, if feasible.

• pillows: Back rests and foam supports can be used to help your patient sit up comfortably. Improvise back rests by using upholstered pillows or wedge-shaped foam rubber.

• bed rails: If your patient tends to fall out of bed (most often young children or the elderly), bed rails can prevent injury. Order bed rails from the surgical supply. Or make your own. Push one side of the bed against a wall. On the other side, line up the backs of chairs for the length of the bed. Keep them in place by topping them with heavy objects such as books.

How to Plug into Services to Help You Pay for Home Care

Facing the trauma of illness can be a tough fight. Dealing with its costs can be a knockout blow. Without question the distractions of home care leave little energy for coping with its financial realities. But they must be faced. And I am convinced that there are uncomplicated ways to do this.

The foundation for paying all home-care costs should be *health insurance coverage*. Most people get health insurance from their employers or professional organizations. Find out if your patient has such coverage. And, if so, what kind? If the policy is gathering dust in a drawer, now is the time to take it out and clear things up. You may discover that the policy contains coverage

for home-health services and other home-care related options
(such as equipment rentals). Suppose the policy seems confusing
to you. Most are baffling to the average person. Call an insurance
agent affiliated with the company that sponsors your patient's
policy. This person can explain the benefits in simple, easy-to-
grasp language. And he or she can offer valuable advice to help
you expand the policy, if necessary.

If your patient doesn't have health insurance, by all means get
some. An excellent source of health insurance information is the
Health Insurance Association of America, 1850 K St., N.W.,
Washington, D.C. 20006. It provides general information about
health insurance and consumer education pamphlets. Furthermore, this organization can help you to judge the reliability of a
particular insurance company and determine which policy may
be best to supplement Medicare coverage.

Tip: Whenever possible try to be involved in a group plan.
These are always less costly than individual policies and their
benefits are often better.

What About Major Medical Insurance?

Your patient needs a policy that will protect against the devastating financial losses of a health catastrophe. You buy major
medical insurance to supplement standard policies that are often
inadequate. Commercial carriers (Equitable, Aetna, etc.) handle
this type of coverage. One important thing: Most major medical
policies do not cover 100% of medical costs. You will be told
you have to pay a *deductible* in the event of illness. That is, you
will have to pay a certain amount of money and the insurance
company will pay the rest. The amount of out-of-pocket funds
you must lay out will depend on the policy you purchase. The
higher the deductible, the less the policy will cost.

Beyond Standard Insurance—
What Are the Alternatives?

Let's start with *health maintenance organizations*. Some employers, instead of offering conventional health insurance, provide an option for HMO's. Or your patient may join one on his or her own. HMO's are groups of doctors and other medical professionals who collaborate to provide total health care for their members on a prepaid basis.

Your patient pays a fee ahead of time and, in the event of illness, surgery, or other medically related conditions, services are rendered—unlimited and any time they are needed. The quality of HMO's varies. If your patient is a member or just thinking of joining, you may get more information by writing the Group Health Association of America, 624 Ninth St. N.W., Washington, D.C., 20001.

Medicare is a health-insurance program for people sixty-five and older and some people under sixty-five, who are disabled or have end-stage renal disease. It's a federal government program run by the Health Care Financing Administration. Medicare has two parts. One is hospital insurance (Part A) and the other is medical insurance (Part B). Medicare is a program with many details that are too numerous to mention here. Your best bet is to consult a social worker or counselor at your local Social Security office to answer to all your questions.

It's worth noting, however, that Medicare does cover some home-health services, such as part-time skilled nursing care, physical therapy, speech therapy, part-time services of home-health aides, medical social services, and medical supplies and equipment provided by home-health agencies participating in the program. (For more information write to the Bureau of Eligibility, Reimbursement and Coverage, Health Care Financing Administration, Rm. 100, East High Rise, 6325 Security Blvd., Baltimore, Md. 21207.) Furthermore, a recent legislative action has provided for unlimited home-health visits; eliminated the three-day prior hospitalization requirement for home-health services under Part A; removed the $75 deductible for home-health services under Part B; and permitted proprietary home-health agencies to participate in states not having licensure laws.

Tip: Medicare can be confusing. A good all-round source of information is *The Medicare Answer Book*, by Gerri Harrington, Harper/Colophon Books, New York, 1982 ($5), at your book store or library.

Medicaid is not the same as Medicare. It's an assistance, not an insurance program. Federal funds are disbursed through the states, and each state designs its own Medicaid procedures. Arizona is the only state without Medicaid. Who is eligible for this aid, which covers an extensive array of home health-care expenses? Certain kinds of needy and low-income people: the aged (sixty-five and over), blind, disabled, members of families with dependent children. Assistance may be given to families whose earnings are inadequate to absorb the cost of extensive medical problems. For information about your patient's eligibility, contact your local welfare department, social worker, or county social services.

Marginal income programs are offered by some states. New York, for example, provides such a program under contract with the New York City Department of Aging and as part of the Older Americans Act Program. Basically this type of service helps to provide homemaker services for people who are just above Medicaid eligibility levels. To find out about the availability of such a program in your area, contact a social worker or county social services office.

Veterans services may provide some money to families of veterans from special funds such as the Soldiers, Sailors and Marine Fund. If you need more information, contact your local veterans administration office.

Private foundations exist to help some needy people and their families. In other words, certain well-to-do individuals have bequeathed money to establish trust funds. The interest earned from these funds is used to help some patients with their medical expenses. Information can be obtained through hospital administration offices or your county social service department.

Ten Care-Giving Hints You Can't Do Without

There's no two ways about it: Care giving is hard emotional and physical work. If you are a care giver, or thinking of becoming one, be sure that you have a realistic idea of home care's major demands. Need some help? The ten hints that follow should answer many of your questions and clarify some of your doubts.

HINT #1: Do You Know What to Expect *During* Home Care?

You should! Meet with your patient's physician *before* home care begins. Get complete information about your patient's condition so that you know the type of care to give—and encounter few (if any!) surprises.

The Home-Care Plan below will help you. Fill it out under the physician's supervision. When completed it will provide you with an accurate picture of your patient's home-care needs.

The Home-Care Plan
1. What is the nature of your patient's condition?
2. Is recovery possible? How long will recovery take?
3. What limitations, if any, will recovery impose on the patient (diet, physical, sexual, social, etc.)?
4. What medications are required (name, desired effects, dosage, frequency, possible side effects, special instructions)?
5. What special treatments are needed?
6. What emergencies may arise from your patient's condition? If emergencies arise, what should be done?
7. What kind of skilled nursing will be needed (visiting nurses, therapists, home-health aides, home attendants, etc.)?

8. What community services, agencies, or religious groups can help with care (Cancer Care, church groups, etc.)?

9. What kinds of special or assistive equipment are needed (wheelchair, cane, hospital bed, etc.)?

10. Additional instructions?

HINT #2: Are You Physically Able to Provide Care?

Consult your physician to be sure that you can handle the rigors of home care. If care-giving jeopardizes your health in any way, find help or another care giver. Don't risk ending up with two sick people in the same house!

HINT #3: Do You View Your Care-Giving Abilities Realistically?

Again and again I have found that too many care givers expect too much from themselves. They say they feel inadequate because they are repelled by certain care tasks, unable to give care twenty-four hours a day, or incapable of making their loved one well. It's natural to want to do as much as you can for someone you love. It's unnatural to work yourself into the ground to do it.

Face reality and your personal limitations. Ask for help from others if you need it. This means that you must delegate some care tasks to family, friends, paid service providers, or volunteers. It also means to ask a friend, physician, nurse, or counselor to listen to you discuss your frustrations and fears. Don't go it alone. If you do you will become emotionally and physically bankrupt.

HINT #4: Have You Put Guilt in Proper Perspective?

Guilt is a sinister sensation that shadows many care givers. If you let yourself, you can feel guilty about everything. You can feel ashamed of not performing medical miracles, of becoming irritable and resentful under care pressures, of not being a good wife, husband, son, etc., of your loved one's being ill and your being well. The list is endless.

The trouble with guilt is that it's tough to camouflage. No matter how hard you try, your patient senses it. And that's an unfair emotional burden to place on anyone.

Try my antidote to guilt: talk. Ventilate your feelings by sharing them with family members and close friends. You may be relieved to know that others feel as you do. If your guilt is intense, or if there is no one to talk to, consult the physician, nurse, or social worker for guidance. They can point you toward professional counseling or support groups for help.

HINT #5: Are You Capable of Maintaining Your Patient's Dignity?

In the world of home care many things can undermine your patient's sense of worth. For instance, loss of independence, loss of certain body functions, changes in body image from surgery or accident, the injustices of the aging process—all can diminish your loved one's sense of self.

That's why it's so important for you to be sensitive to your patient's feelings. You have the power to create an atmosphere of acceptance and reassurance. Try loving words, warm touches, embraces—and listening. Without question people heal faster in supportive and caring environments.

HINT #6: Can You Be an Advocate for Your Patient?

Advocates stand up for the rights and needs of their patients. Case in point: During some home-care visits that I made with a visiting nurse I observed that one forty-year-old man with diabetes always put on his best face for us. Yet the moment the nurse stepped out of the room, his expression folded into sadness and discomfort. Finally, I told the nurse about the man's dual personality. She said, "That happens a lot. A doctor or nurse must know the whole picture about a patient. Family members should speak up for their patients and when necessary tell medical professionals exactly what's going on."

HINT #7: Do You Have a Sense of Humor?

I hope so. Because so much of home care's success depends on attitude. You can let the difficulties of caring for a loved one drag you down. Or you can neutralize them by finding humor in moments that can be otherwise frustrating.

One young woman who was caring for her mother—a victim of cancer *and* a mental breakdown—told me: "My mother's condition was gruesome. I didn't know what to do first—mourn her illness or grieve because she had a break with reality. For weeks I was deeply depressed. I eventually realized that if I didn't change my tune I'd be a goner. So slowly I tried to find the lighter side of things. One day my mother, whose illness had transformed her into a chronic complainer, consented to taking a walk outdoors. I had been coaxing her to do this for weeks. I went to her room to pick her up only to find her sitting at the edge of the bed with her head in her hands. 'What's the matter now, Mother?' I asked. She looked at me and said, 'I can't go. I don't have anything attractive to wear.' Only weeks before, her comment would have made me want to pull the covers over my head. This time I laughed at the irony—and took joy that for the first time in months she was concerned about her appearance."

Along these lines, consider reading Norman Cousins's book, *Anatomy of an Illness as Perceived by the Patient: Reflections on Healing and Regeneration*. Cousins made an amazing recovery from a serious illness which he attributes to the powerful force of positive emotions—and large doses of laughter. His book has been an inspiration to many. Try it!

HINT #8: Do You Know How to Be the Physician's Care Partner?

In most cases the physician will rely on you for information about the patient's condition and progress. To be sure that you get the most important points across quickly and clearly, remember to:

• be prepared. Have all the information you need about the patient in front of you before you speak. This is especially helpful during phone conversations. Fill index cards with your questions or exact information.

• place events *in the order* they happened. Describe your loved one's condition. To illustrate: "My husband had pain in his chest after dinner, this morning he looked pale, this afternoon he was dizzy," is not as helpful as: "This morning my husband looked pale, he felt dizzy this afternoon, and after dinner he complained of chest pains."

• provide details. Don't speak in generalities. "My mother didn't feel well today," is not as good as: "My mother was nauseated and had a severe headache today."

HINT #9: Is It Possible to Handle the Noncommunicative Physician?

You bet. But it takes a bit of know-how and some confidence. Recognize these telltale signs: aloofness, reluctance to answer your questions, responses in technical jargon that are difficult to understand. It is important to remember the following:

• You have the right to receive answers to your questions.

• Your deserve clear explanations.

• You are paying for a service and should expect cooperation, and respect. Don't tolerate a condescending or patronizing manner.

My advice: Be assertive. When you don't understand something, request (diplomatically) an immediate explanation in language you can handle. If the physician is a cool number who keeps you at a distance, persist. More often than not a gentle pursuit of the facts will get you the answers you need.

However, if your physician is constantly difficult to talk to, is condescending or uncooperative, consider changing doctors.

HINT #10: Beware of Physicians Who Hold Back Information

During my home-care travels for this book I met a sixty-year-old woman who had had a hysterectomy, mastectomy, and removal of her adrenal glands. All this was done to help "fight" the cancer that was clearly taking over her system.

While speaking to her family I discovered that they were unaware of the seriousness of the woman's condition. Sometime later a nurse on the case told me the reason for this: The physician had withheld important facts about the patient's health. He had *not* told the family that the woman had only a few months to live. He had provided no warnings about the medical emergencies that could arise from her failing condition. Shocked, I soon learned that although this physician's behavior is not the norm, it's also not unusual. Why do doctors hold back information? Some prejudge a person's ability to understand or cope with certain facts. Some physicians pick up signals that read "I don't want to know anything bad." Still others may have difficulty being the bearers of tragic news, so they avoid touching on it altogether.

Why am I telling you this? Because as care giver you *should know everything* about your patient's condition so you can be prepared for all situations—especially those health crises that can occur when patients have chronic or deteriorating illnesses.

The bottom line: As care giver you must be able to handle full disclosure about your patient's health—no matter what the prognosis.

Home-Care Helpers:
The Latest Programs
to Make Home Care Easier

By now you probably picture home care as a health plan that exists totally within the home setting. For many patients that's an accurate assessment. But for a growing number of people health-care services are received outside the home on a day to day basis.

Here's a sampling of these programs. Perhaps one will meet your loved one's special needs.

Adult Day Care Programs:

These are day-care programs for health services in an ambulatory setting designed for people who don't need twenty-four-hour institutional care and yet because of physical or mental impairments are not capable of full-time independent living.

Participants are referred to the program by their physicians or other sources, such as institutional discharge planning programs or other social service agencies.

Adult day care aims to maintain and restore health. In the process it offers participants opportunities to socialize and thereby overcome the isolation so often associated with chronic or debilitating illnesses. Generally, these programs provide a wide assortment of services, including nursing, nutrition counseling, physical/speech/occupational therapies, physical examinations, meals, and more. There are programs in progress and development around the country. For more information write: Health Care Financing Administration, Health Standards and Quality Bureau, 1849 Gwynn Oak Ave., Baltimore, Md. 21207. (See Chapter 12.)

Cooperative Care Programs:

These programs are based on an innovative and most attractive idea. New York University Medical Center was the first institution to start a co-op care program. Under its auspices, patients recovering from surgery or disabling or chronic illnesses reside in a setting that strives to be as un-hospitallike as possible. Patient education is emphasized, as patients are taught how to care for themselves at home, prepare meals according to prescribed diets, and rethink the unhealthy life-styles that got them into trouble. In addition, a close family member is encouraged to stay with the patient (often overnight) to learn how to help him or her in the home setting. The NYU Hospital project is the first of this type. Plans are under way in Portland, Oregon, to get a similar program going. Others are projected for development throughout the country. For more information write: New York University Medical Center, Public Information, 560 First Ave., New York, N.Y. 10016.

Social Health Maintenance Organizations:

The Metropolitan Jewish Geriatric Center in Brooklyn, New York, has started a project that intends to provide comprehensive services for both well and impaired senior citizens. It is a demonstration program designed to provide a full range of in-patient, ambulatory, rehabilitative, home-health, and personal support services within a set budget. It is hoped that this program, through better case management, will help reduce the amount of inappropriate services and the high expenses that are often associated with health-care delivery for the elderly. Demonstration programs along these lines are being developed around the country in places such as Portland, Oregon, Long Beach, California, and Minneapolis, Minnesota. Contact the U.S. Health Care Financing Administration in Baltimore, Maryland, for information about experimental programs that may be in your area.

3

Your Bible
for Home-Care Tasks

This chapter is designed to give you explicit instructions for many of the home-care tasks you will face. Of course, you may have additional questions. They should be addressed to the physician or nurse.

Home-Care Basic #1:
How to Keep the Sickroom Spotless

Naturally, you must keep the sickroom clean. After all, a sanitary sickroom protects the patient—and you—from unnecessary contamination. And an orderly room is simply a nice place to stay.

You'll find it easier to maintain your patient's room if you:

• wash your hands before and after patient contact

• clean furnishings and surfaces with warm water, soap, and disinfectant (Lysol, Pinesol, etc.)

• remove dust and dirt with a damp cloth; vacuum floor or carpet

• prevent spread of infection from contagious patients by using disposable cups, dishes, and eating utensils

• transport cleaning equipment or patient supplies from room to room by cart. Any light, easy-to-move furniture on wheels will do. You can adapt a rolling coffee table or bar. Or try a chair on wheels. Simply use the seat as a tabletop and push. A box may be used to hold supplies and to prevent them from falling off the chair.

A word about flowers and plants...and other harborers of germs: They may be pretty to look at, but they provide fertile ground for bacterial growth—a potential health hazard. So bear the following in mind.

• Plants and flowers should not be left soaking in stagnant water. Change it daily to prevent foul smells and bacterial growth.

• Dead plants and flowers should be disposed of immediately; they breed germs.

• Room fresheners or deodorants can diminish sickroom odors. To avoid odors, clean waste basket daily, discard all soiled dressings and body wastes.

• Humidifiers or vaporizers containing pans of water should be changed daily to prevent bacteria growth and mildew.

How to Remove the Most Common Home-Care Stains

• feces: Soak fabric in cold water. Rinse, then wash with soap and hot water. Use brush to scrub out stain.

• urine: Soak fabric in boiling water. Pour 5% Lysol solution over it. Rinse in warm water.

• blood: Clean as soon as you can. Soak fabric in cold water. If fabric is white use a little ammonia. When stain is brown, wash with warm water and soap.

• iodine: Clean soiled fabric as soon as possible. Pour hot water onto stain. For old stain use bleach. Rinse in warm, soapy water.

Home-Care Basic #2:
How to Keep Your Patient Comfortably Dressed

Your patient will be most comfortable in cotton garments that are nonrestricting. Common sense will tell you to provide pajamas or nightgown, nonslip slippers, bed jacket or a robe.

You can make an inexpensive home-care gown for your patient. Take an old man-tailored shirt (a woman's shirt may be used for a child) and cut off the collar, cuffs, and button panels—if the weather is warm, you may want to cut the sleeves short. Then sew several snaps in to keep garment secure. The shirt should be worn loosely and be easy to remove. *Or*, use an oversized cotton T-shirt so that its bottom comes at least mid-thigh to knee-length on the patient. This is a comfortable alternative. *Or*, you can purchase a ready-made hospital gown at a surgical supply.

Home-Care Basic #3: Surefire Rest and Exercise Tips

Nothing can beat home care for restfulness. No hospital noises or strict schedules. No roommate chatter or institutional racket. You can enhance the recuperative environment by supplying your patient with extra blankets and pillows for comfort; keeping bedpans and urinals in easy reach; keeping household noise and commotion to a minimum; instructing telephone callers to restrict their well wishes to the patient's awake time.

Sleep

Sleep needs differ from person to person. For some, normal sleep lasts between six and nine hours. For others it is less. Eight hours is average.

Your patient's need for sleep will depend on his or her condition, the treatment received, and sleep habits before illness. Ask the physician to determine the amount of sleep required for your patient to recover and maintain health.

Insomnia

This is the inability to obtain normal sleep. It may mean trouble falling or staying asleep. Many people who complain of sleeplessness often underestimate the amount of sleep they have actually had. So if your patient complains of insomnia, observe periodically during the night to doublecheck. Consult the physician if you have any uncertainties.

What causes insomnia during home care? Pain, medication side effects, noise, type of illness, anxiety, depression, uncomfortable room temperature, fever, overeating, frequent urination, hunger, extreme fatigue are all possibilities. Certainly, any sleep problems lasting more than two nights should be reported to the physician. But before you determine insomnia is a problem, be sure your loved one's life is not filled with "insomnia inducers." Caffeine is the most common. Avoid serving caffeinated coffee, tea, and soft drinks. Chocolate and cocoa have a caffeinelike substance, too. Also, discourage these stimulating activities before bed: watching exciting television, listening to fast-paced music, reading exciting stories, vigorous exercise, and eating a heavy meal.

Touch

During my research for this book I met many home-care patients and their families. The patients who seemed calmest and most serene were those who received regular doses of touch. Not surprisingly, research shows that people who are *rarely* touched frequently feel increased levels of anxiety.

Don't be afraid to use touch liberally. Warmly stroke your patient's arm, gently caress the face. Sit close to the patient. Even the subtle pressure of your hand during moments of silence can communicate support and love far better than words.

There are some patients to whom touch is especially beneficial. Your patient may fall in one of these groups:

• patients who feel isolated because of communication difficulties

• patients who have had disfiguring surgery or accident (touch can boost self-esteem)

• patients who are emotionally disturbed (anxious, depressed, confused).

Touch can help maintain contact with someone who is "difficult to reach."

The Good Word About Massage

A massage can feel like magic. It manipulates the body's soft tissues, offering mild exercise, and in the process relaxing the recipient. It is also a nonthreatening form of touch. I believe in the efficacy of massage as good medicine. I'm not suggesting that it's a cure-all. Rather, when used properly and appropriately it can be a delightful contact that communicates your caring and love to the patient.

You can perform a body massage at home. Or you can just massage one body part at a time. For example, take your patient's hand. Put some moisturizing cream on the flat part of your fingers, start at your loved one's fingertips and gently stroke toward the heart. You can use the same technique on the foot. This type of contact can be both nonthreatening and comforting. If you'd like to learn more about massage, its therapeutic as well as emotional benefits, read *The Massage Book*, by George Downing (Random House, New York, 1982), at your library or bookstore. This publication offers detailed but simple instructions for giving massage.

Remember the following caveats about massage.

• Never massage a patient who is in pain.

• Never massage a patient who has had recent wounds, infections, hemorrhages, hypertension, or clotting disorders.

• Never massage a patient who feels threatened or anxious about it.

• Always get the physician's permission before massaging your patient.

Exercise

The decision for exercise and activity for your patient should be made in collaboration with the physician. If your patient has a short-term illness, mobility during personal-care tasks such as toileting and bathing may be sufficient. However, disabled or long-term patients may need special exercise plans such as range-of-motion exercises, physical therapy, occupational therapy, and so on. Ask the physician or nurse for guidance.

Home-Care Basic #4:
The Last Word on Hot and Cold Therapies

Heat

Heat raises the temperature of the specific part or area of the body to which it is applied. It is often used to lessen pain and muscle stiffness. It may also be administered to prepare certain patients for the movements of physical therapy.

Some time ago I used a heating pad for a pulled back muscle. I stayed on that pad for hours waiting for miracles. None came for a very simple reason few people know: The greatest benefit from the application of local heat is often reached in twenty minutes. After that no further local elevation of temperature can be achieved. The increased blood flow to the area simply carries the heat away to the whole body.

The bottom line: If you intend to apply heat, do it for *only twenty minutes at a time*. Beyond that, be cautious when applying heat to a patient who has experienced a sensation loss. The inability to judge proper temperature can lead to serious skin burns.

Home-Heat Therapies

Here's a brief glossary of therapies to let you know what the physician or therapist has in mind when a particular one is prescribed: *hydrocollator packs* (sophisticated heating pads made from canvas and filled with silica gel that can be contoured to fit the body); *infra-red heat* (infra-red lamps that radiate heat onto a specific body area); *paraffin bath* (used to ease the painfulness in joints of the hands of arthritis sufferers. Paraffin wax is placed inside a special container where it's heated until melted. Patients dip their hands or feet into the bath for relief); *ultrasound* (high-frequency waves that penetrate the body's tissue to apply a unique deep heat); *whirlpool* (patient places a body part into a tub of water. The water is whirled around by a strong motor creating a massaging sensation; used to ease joint pain and discomfort from fractures).

Cold

The use of cold therapy is most often done with a large ice cube or pack of ice cubes. The physician may prescribe cold therapy to reduce swelling, spasticity, or inflammation.

In most cases you will be told to rub the ice or place it over the affected area until your patient feels some numbness. Expect this to take about fifteen minutes or a bit less. You will need to know how long to apply the ice without harming the patient. Ask the physician for explicit instructions as each patient's needs are unique. Warning: Patients who have a sensation loss on the affected area may need special care. Do not apply cold therapy until you have consulted the physician.

Home-Care Basic #5: Everything You Need to Know to Prevent Pressure Sores

Meet the bane of the bedridden and immobilized patient's existence: Pressure sores (also called bedsores and decubitus ulcers) are skin ulcers that appear when parts of the body are compressed by lying or sitting down (see Figure 3). Even the persistent weight of bedding and bedclothes can lead to sores.

Why should you care? Because sores can start within days of immobilization. And once they do, they're tough to cure. Neglected ones are not only painful, but they can become infected, require hospitalization, and—in severe cases—cause death.

Pressure-Sore Alert

Watch out for spots of red, shiny skin that lack sensation. This is the first sign of skin breakdown. Treat by washing, then lubricating the area according to physician's advice. Protect the "early" sore with skin shields (see below). Reposition your patient so there is no more pressure on vulnerable spots.

Call physician or nurse *immediately* if redness leads to opening, peeling, or a break in the skin.

High-Risk Patients

Some people are more susceptible to pressure sores than others. Your patient may fall into one of these categories:
- long-term bedridden or wheelchair-bound patients
- elderly and immobilized or bedridden
- patients with poor circulation
- diabetics
- incontinent patients
- patients wearing appliances, bandages, or traction devices
- patients who cannot manage proper hygiene
- patients with sensation losses.

How to Prevent Pressure Sores

- Be sure that your loved one moves frequently. Do not allow him or her to stay in the same position for more than two hours. Assist to new position if necessary. Wheelchair patients should shift weight from one side to another every fifteen minutes.
- Supervise proper hygiene. Daily bathing stimulates skin and prevents skin breakdown. Focus on bony prominences such as hips, elbows, heels, ankles, etc.
- Bathe incontinent patients after each episode.
- If your patient's wheelchair-bound, watch skin areas that fall against the chair. Clean, stimulate, and protect them daily.

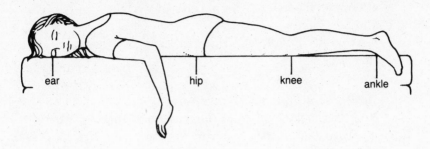

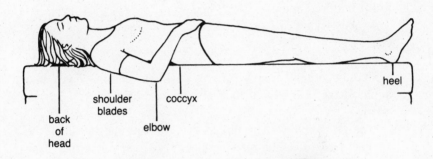

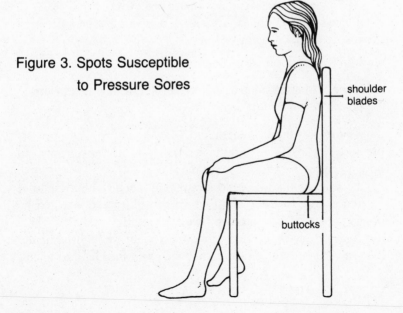

Figure 3. Spots Susceptible to Pressure Sores

• Remove food crumbs from bed and wrinkled sheets. They can irritate skin.

• Avoid harsh detergents that can leave an irritating residue on the fabric.

Devices that Prevent Pressure Sores

You can purchase the following at surgical supply stores.

1. Sheep skin, Kodel, synthetic fur pads; can be sized to fit area; attached with adhesive tape or Velcro strap.

2. Commercial heel and elbow protectors.

3. Rubber air rings; can be slipped under your patient's bottom to lift buttocks and coccyx off bed.

4. Air, water, and other specialty mattresses. Consult physician or nurse for advice.

Or you can make your own.

• cotton donut: Take strips of absorbent cotton. Twist into donut shape. Close with adhesive tape. Place under heels or elbow.

• no-pressure box: This device lifts blankets and sheets off the patient. Get a medium size cardboard box and cut in the shape of a table (see Figure 4). Place under bed covers.

• flannel material (blanket, sheets): Wrap around pressure-sensitive spot or place against area.

Home-Care Basic #6: Movement and Your Patient

In most cases movement is good medicine. It maintains muscle tone, promotes bone strength and joint flexibility, and prevents pressure sores. Ask the physician or nurse which movements and how much are best for your patient.

One technique you should know more about is the Range of Motion exercises. They are used for bedridden and wheelchair-bound patients. There are two types: (1) *passive* exercises which use another person to help move the patient through particular motions; (2) *active* exercises which are performed by the patient.

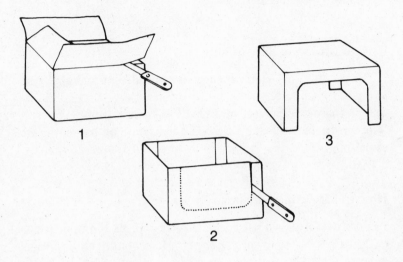

Figure 4. No-Pressure Box

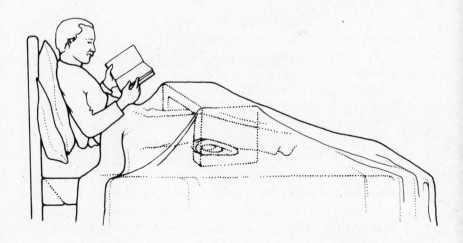

I suggest that you ask a nurse or physical therapist to instruct you in the movements that are most suited to your patient. Then you can do them regularly on your own.

How to Move the Sick Infant

1. Ask the physician or nurse for specific instructions pertaining to your baby.
2. Important: Infants' neck muscles aren't well-developed. Support the head. Make sure head and body are moved at the same time.

How to Move the Bedridden Patient

Your best bet is to ask medical professionals for guidance as each patient has very special needs. Meanwhile, here are some general guidelines that you can apply in all situations.

1. Always maintain a healthy moving posture. Stand erect with knees bent slightly, feet flat and apart, toes pointed in the direction of movement.
2. Tell your loved one what you intend to do so that you can get as much cooperation as possible.
3. Avoid lifting your patient whenever possible. Instead, roll, pivot, or slide the person toward you.
4. Ask the patient to help as much as his or her condition allows.
5. Always put the bulk of weight on your legs—not your back.
6. Be alert! Stop if you are hurting the patient.
7. Always get help when moving a large or heavy person.
8. Wear low-heeled shoes.

Tip: If your patient is bedridden or immobilized and you must move him or her, *get professional instruction*. A visiting nurse or home-health aide can come to the home just once to show you exactly what to do. Learning moving techniques from a professional person is far better and safer than simply reading about them.

How to Slide the Supine Patient Toward You

1. If you have any back problems consult your physician before moving the patient.
2. Slide both your hands (palms up, close together) under the patient's legs just below the knees.
3. Pull legs toward you.
4. Slide both your hands under patient's hips.
5. Pull patient toward you.
6. Slide your arms under patient's shoulders so head is on your forearm. Hold patient's shoulders with your hand.
7. Hold patient's neck with your other hand. Pull individual toward you.

How to Move Your Patient to a Chair

1. Select chair of convenient height. Place chair alongside bed to make distance from bed to chair as short as possible.
2. Ask the patient or assist patient to sit up at edge of bed.
3. Stand directly opposite patient, keep your feet together with your knees slightly bent. Slide your arms under patient's armpits, brace your knees against the patient's, and pivot from bed to chair.
4. Keep close tabs on patient sitting in chair. Your physician or nurse can prescribe a device to help your patient sit upright, if necessary.

How to Move the Helpless Patient Up in Bed

1. Move bed away from wall with enough space for you to stand. Remove pillows. Lie patient flat.
2. If bed has wheels, lock them; if hospital bed, be sure it's in a flat position.

3. Stand behind the head of the bed. It may be easier if you stand on a small stool.

4. Lean over head of bed. Reach over patient's shoulders and lock your arms under patient's armpits. Ask patient to assist as much as he or she can by bending knees and pushing with feet.

5. Pull patient up. (Important: At the slightest discomfort stop activity immediately and get help.)

How to Help the Cooperative Patient Move Up in Bed

1. Be sure that bed is flat. Remove all pillows.

2. Stand alongside the bed near your patient's weakest side. You should face the head of the bed with your feet apart, one foot in front of the other. Bend your knees slightly.

3. Place your arm nearest the bed under your patient's armpit.

4. Ask the patient to take his or her stronger arm and grasp the top of the bed. While in that position the stronger leg should be bent.

5. In a coordinated movement your patient should pull with his or her arm and dig in the heel of the stronger leg while you lift your loved one up in bed.

How to Help Your Patient Sit Up in Bed

1. Sit on the edge of the patient's bed close to the level of his or her shoulders.

2. Make sure your feet are flat and spaced apart for balance. Lift with your legs, not with your back!

3. Slide your arms under patient's closest shoulder. For example, slip your right arm under his or her right shoulder.

4. Lift patient and slide pillows or bedrest to prop up your loved one.

Tips for Moving the Frail, Elderly, Post-Surgical or Injured Patient

• Avoid abrupt movements. They can frighten some patients.

• Be sensitive to your patient's discomfort. For example, movement for some arthritic patients may hurt. Slow the pace as your patient requires.

• If moving causes discomfort at the wound site or adjacent area (post-surgery), have the patient hold a pillow pressed against the incision. This is called splinting and should alleviate most discomfort.

• If patient has had an injury or broken bone, be sure that you don't put pressure on the sensitive area.

Moving Tips for You, the Care Giver

Do not move the patient by yourself if:

• you have back problems
• the patient is obese
• you have had recent surgery
• the patient's condition demands that he or she be moved in total alignment by two carriers
• you have *any* difficulty.

If patient experiences pain during movement, ask physician if a painkiller can be administered prior to movement to make things easier. If the physician says yes, know that some painkillers may create "confusion states" in susceptible patients. Be sure to give your patient close attention and support during all movement to prevent falls and other accidents.

Home-Care Basic #7: How to Turn Bathing into a Health-Giving Therapy

Bathing isn't just for cleansing your patient. It's also an opportunity for you to observe your loved one carefully; a time to spot bruises, bleeding, rashes, skin breakdown or discharges. The simple body movements of soaping, rinsing, and repositioning can provide light exercise and stimulate circulation. And as you wash your patient with long, gentle strokes you are providing soothing and comforting contact.

How often should you bathe your patient? Frankly, it's best to check with the doctor to find out how much bathing is wise, because bathing can be too much of a good thing. In excess it can tire the unwell individual and lead to dry skin. On the other hand, there are body parts that must be washed every day to prevent infection and pressure sores. They are: face, underarms, genitals, rectal area, all bony prominences, especially elbows, heels, lower back, spine, hips, and buttocks.

Bath alert! Don't bathe patients who:

• are in severe pain and find that the movement of bathing adds to discomfort. A partial bedbath is an alternative.

• have stitches. Get permission from the physician.

• wear casts. Take precaution to avoid wetting cast (see Home-Care Basic #8).

• are elderly and have dry skin. Avoid excessive bathing. Lubricate skin with body lotion or moisturizer after bath.

• have mobility problems unless special assistive devices have been provided such as handrails around the tub.

How to Provide Mouth Care for the Helpless Patient

The easiest way to handle oral hygiene in this type of situation: Gather equipment at bedside including toothbrush, toothpaste, glass of cool water, small basin or container, dental floss, towel, and mouthwash (optional). Wash your hands thoroughly.

When patient has difficulty keeping his or her mouth open, avoid placing your fingers in the mouth to open it (you risk a human bite which can be dangerous). Instead, hold the patient's mouth open with the cloth-covered handle of a spoon. Encourage patient to do as much brushing as possible. If he or she needs help, open the mouth, moisten brush, and apply paste. Brush as you would your own teeth. Of course, patient must rinse into container.

Tip: If your loved one cannot tolerate a toothbrush because of sensitivity inside the mouth, improvise with cotton swab. Dip it into a solution of half hydrogen peroxide and half water. Swab teeth, tongue, and gums. Ask patient to rinse. If that's impossible take a clean swab. Dip it in clean water and reswab mouth surfaces. Wash your hands thoroughly. Another option is the Toothette. This is a commercially-made premoistened, mint-flavored applicator. It can clean and soothe teeth and gums—without rinsing. And, it's disposable. For more information write: Halbrand, Inc., Willoughby, Ohio, 44094, or check your surgical supply store.

The Bed Bath

The bed bath comes in handy when your patient cannot take a regular bath or shower. There's the *dry bed bath*, which is simple but should *not* be done every day. Gently rub body lotion on your patient's body (not on mucous membranes). This will lubricate the skin, preventing dryness and skin breakdown. You may want to alternate this one with the wet one to help avoid excessive bathing.

The *wet bed bath* is a true body wash. I suggest that you ask your patient to bathe as much of him- or herself as possible. This fosters independence and makes your job lots easier. Just remember not to rush the patient as that only adds unnecessary tension. Baths should be taken more often if your patient perspires heavily.

How to Give a Bed Bath

1. Adjust the thermostat so that the room is at a comfortable temperature. Ensure *total* privacy.

2. Gather equipment at bedside: warm basin of water, two washcloths, bath towels, soap, body lotion and/or deodorant, bed clothes.

3. As your patient disrobes be sure that he or she is never totally undressed. Cover with large bath towel or robe.

4. Protect bedding by placing a large towel under the patient.

5. Take one body area at a time and clean. Try this order: arms and hands, face and ears, neck, chest, abdomen. Using second washcloth and fresh basin of water, cleanse neck, back, underarms, navel. Whenever possible ask the patient to wash own genitals and rectal area.

6. Watch out for skin abnormalities (irritation, tenderness, breakdown, etc.)

7. Change water. Wash legs and feet. Dry.

8. Have you missed these often missed spots: corners of eyes, inside ears, under women's breasts, between toes, female genitals (wash front to back), male genitals (wash alongside scrotum)?

9. Make sure patient is totally dry. Then apply deodorant or light dusting of talcum powder.

10. Have patient put on fresh bedclothes.

What You Must Know About Bathing a Diabetic's Feet

So many home-care patients have diabetes that I could not write this chapter without addressing their very special needs. The bottom line here is that diabetes often interferes with the circulation of blood in legs and feet. Therefore, any opening in the surface of the skin, infection, or irritation can be slow to heal. In some patients this can threaten health. To avoid problems that could lead to serious infection and in severe cases, amputation, be sure to:

• wash feet daily with mild soap and lukewarm water. Never let them soak. Never use hot water.

• dry feet with a clean towel after washing. Dry thoroughly between toes.

• check feet daily. Note the soles, between the toes. Look for pus, swelling, sores, cracks, redness. Call physician immediately if any appear.

• keep foot skin soft by lubricating it daily with a small amount of body lotion. Don't put lotion between toes.

• do keep sweating feet dry with talcum powder.

• be careful when cutting toenails. Avoid nicking skin. Never trim nails shorter than ends of toes. Only a podiatrist should cut nails!

• Never tear off dead skin around calluses or use commercial removers.

The Tub Bath

During a recent visit to an occupational therapist I was amazed to see the equipment she had to make tub bathing easier and safer for many home-care patients. There were tub rails to grab on to, hydraulic lifts to pick the patient up and put him into the tub, nonslip mats and adhesive tape attached to the tub's bottom to prevent accidents, bath seats to sit on, and so on. Check a surgical supply catalogue for ideas or consult a medical professional.

If your patient can handle a tub bath, it's important to encourage him or her to be as independent as possible. Try to allow complete privacy. Be sure to keep the bathroom door unlocked or slightly ajar and stay within earshot in case your patient needs help. Never leave a very young child, elderly person, confused patient, or depressed patient alone in the tub.

If your patient uses a wheelchair, propel the chair to the tub's edge so legs can be brought over the side. Lock brakes and hold chair steady. Ask patient to slide into tub. Assist and support if necessary. When the patient returns to the chair, hold it steady as he or she slides backward into the seat.

Tub Accident Alert: Fainting in the Tub

What do you do if your patient faints in the tub? Support his or her head and shoulders. Let out all the water. Cover your patient with anything handy (towel, robe, etc.). If patient is too heavy to lift out of tub, call for assistance.

A Few Words About Showers

You may find that a shower is easier to manage than tub bathing. Certainly, patients who preferred showers before illness may still want them.

Prevent accidents by using a nonslip mat or tape on the shower floor. Also, shower chairs can be life-savers for patients who are shaky on their feet. Purchase them at the surgical supply store. Or improvise by using a small metal or plastic chair that you may have at home.

How to Give a Soothing Sponge Bath

This is a wonderful way to comfort and relax your loved one. Use it to refresh the feverish, perspiring, or tense person. It does not require the preparation and paraphernalia of a bed bath. Just fill a basin with comfortably warm water—don't use soap. Then ask your patient to remove his or her pajamas and put on a robe. Expose one body part at a time and, using a washcloth or sponge, bathe the body leisurely. Long strokes are the best. Focus on the back, neck, and face. When you're finished, dry the patient thoroughly.

Shampooing a Patient's Hair in Bed

This is not only possible, but with the purchase of some inexpensive equipment, it's easy.

You will need waterproof protection for the bed. An old vinyl shower curtain, plastic tablecloth or the like will do. Surgical supply stores offer inflatable shampoo basins and shower trays. Both are designed to hold the patient's head, allowing for in-bed washing. Also use two bath towels, shampoo, pitcher of water, and, in case of spills, floor protection such as plastic covering or newspapers.

1. Adjust bed to a comfortable work height. Be sure the room is at a comfortable temperature.

2. Place your patient's head on shampoo tray or basin. Cover shoulders with a towel. (You can make patient's head lower than shoulders by placing a small towel under them.)

3. Pour water onto patient's hair. Apply shampoo and lather up. Rinse as often as necessary.

4. The trick is to work quickly so that you don't fatigue or chill your patient.

5. When finished, dry hair with blow dryer.

Tip: Tangled hair is a drag to comb out. Save a lot of elbow-grease by combing out the tangle in small sections. Hold small section of hair above the tangle point. Comb out with downward strokes. Slowly unsnarl hair. Patients with long hair can diminish tangles by wearing pony tails or braids.

Home-Care Basic #8: Cast Care That's Foolproof

Physicians apply plaster casts to keep particular body parts in proper position. Casts are placed on arms, ankles, legs, and larger body areas such as hips or abdomen. They are even applied to broken bones after some surgeries.

Skin-Care Savvy for Cast Wearers

• If skin under cast itches *do not* stick anything inside cast to scratch—especially if there are stitches. Watch children to make sure they do not stick foreign objects inside casts. Tip: Tap on the cast over the itching. Use a blunt instrument. Or you can blow air inside with a bulb syringe.

• Cast edges sometimes irritate skin. Ease this problem by padding them with cotton, sheepskin, flannel, etc. Make sure this material does not slip inside cast.

• Cleanse area around cast daily. Avoid wetting cast.

• Massage areas around cast often with alcohol. Don't use lotion or creams around or inside cast. They are sticky and can leave an irritating residue.

Cast-Care Don'ts

• Don't put pressure on a wet cast.

• Don't get cast wet. Use plastic bags or other waterproof coverings in wet weather and while bathing or showering. Commercial cast protectors are available at surgical supply stores.

• Don't fret about a dirty cast. You can use white shoe polish to brighten it. Important: Use a little polish, as too much will dampen and soften cast.

The Seven Most Common Cast Problems— And What to Do About Them

1. Swelling. If this happens after activity, elevate your patient's limb. Persistent swelling needs immediate medical attention.

2. Sensation abnormalities. Your patient should have feeling in all parts of the limb, fingers, and toes. Pain, numbness, or tingling are significant causes for concern. Call physician.

3. Odors. Generally, casts don't smell, but sometimes foods or liquids spilled inside them can cause odors. More important are odors emerging from casts covering wounds. This is serious and may mean infection at the wound site. Call physician, at once.

4. Discharge. Another serious sign. Call physician immediately.

5. Loss of movement. Has your patient experienced loss of movement in fingers or toes? If so, call physician.

6. Pain. Any increase in pain or onset of new pain should receive prompt medical attention.

7. Circulation. Detect circulation problems by squeezing fingers and toes. They should appear white when squeezed and redden when released. If this fails to happen, call physician.

Home-Care Basic #9: The Most Efficient Way to Care for Your Patient's Most Intimate Routines

Illness has a way of interfering with a person's ability to eliminate wastes. Your patient may have difficulty voiding or defecating. This may be due to disease, prolonged bed rest, or post-surgical procedures, even medication side effects. True, toileting is one of the most inelegant sides of home care. But it's a necessity, and in this section I will show you how to make it as simple for you and your patient as possible.

There are some important things you should always remember.

• Beware of the adult patient who is able to use the bathroom—yet feigns helplessness. If allowed, this person can become overly dependent on you, and that can be emotionally and physically exhausting. Gently insist that your loved one be as independent as possible.

• Never show disgust when toileting your patient. If you find some aspects of toilet-care difficult, ask other family members, friends, or medical professionals for help.

• Use toileting as a time to check your patient's skin for abnormalities. Also, note the characteristics of stool and urine (see Chapter 5).

Bedpans

They are portable, plastic toilet seats made of plastic, rubber, or steel. They can save a trip to the bathroom. Just slide one under your patient's bottom.

There are two types: *regular*, the most commonly used, and *fracture*. Fracture bedpans are easier to slide under immobile or obese patients. Purchase at the surgical supply store.

How to Use a Bedpan

The secret of successful bedpan use is to offer it to your patient *frequently*. Some patients, reluctant to bother their care givers, may hold in urine or bowel movements, causing additional health problems. Be alert and sensitive to this possibility.

Once your patient is atop the bedpan (you may have to assist!) allow him or her total privacy. Please don't stand there waiting for "something to happen."

If your patient's bottom sticks to the bedpan due to perspiration or incontinence solve the problem by dusting the bedpan surface with talcum powder.

When toileting is finished, make certain that your patient's genital and rectal areas are washed and completely dry. This is a safeguard against irritation, skin breakdown, and urinary tract infections.

What should you do if your patient says, "I can't void on the bedpan"? You can sometimes nudge nature by placing your patient's hand in a dish of water, or allowing running water to be heard from a nearby faucet. Important: The inability to urinate *may be* a serious physical problem brought on by side effects of certain medications and other underlying conditions. If it persists for more than twelve hours, call your physician.

Bedridden or wheelchair-bound males may have an easier time voiding into a urinal than a bedpan. Urinals can be purchased at a drugstore, surgical supply—or improvised at home. Simply use an empty milk or juice carton, cut off the top of the carton to allow access and wash after use. These may be reused.

Bedside Commodes

These are portable toilets that resemble a small chair. There is a container underneath the seat to catch urine and fecal matter.

A person can slide from the bed onto the commode. I met one woman who transformed her storebought commode into a show piece by sewing a lovely floral cover for it. To the untrained eye it looked like a piece of upholstered furniture rather than an appliance for toileting. Commodes are ideal for long-term patients who cannot make it to the bathroom, and for small children who can be carried to and fro. Purchase at surgical supply.

Incontinence—How to Cope and Maintain Your Loved One's Dignity

Incontinence means that a patient has lost bladder and/or bowel control. This can be caused by disease, drug side effects, emotional factors, surgery, or loss of muscle tone, especially in the elderly.

Imagine how you would feel if you urinated or defecated involuntarily, and you'll get some idea of what the incontinent patient experiences. It can be embarrassing, even traumatic. Your loved one may feel burdensome to you, not "whole," or afraid that health is deteriorating. Ease your patient's fears by showing compassion and understanding. Above all, don't reprimand the incontinent patient for something he or she cannot help. Instead provide reassurance. Comments such as these may be helpful: "The doctor said that this will happen because of surgery, medication, etc. It's natural under these circumstances. Please don't worry." Or if the patient is embarrassed, you may say something like: "This is *not* a problem for me. But I will ask the doctor if something can be done to change this situation."

I believe that the best way to deal with incontinence is to *prevent accidents* before they happen, and if they do occur to correct them as quickly as possible. How?

• Provide a bedpan or urinal frequently so that the patient is not likely to retain urine until it can be held no longer.

• Never bring attention to a person's incontinence by making

him or her wear demeaning clothing such as a diaper. Diapering
is demoralizing to anyone but an infant. Even an obvious absorbent pad placed directly underneath the patient is an ever
present reminder of the problem.

Tip: Insert a Chux pad to absorb urine (purchase at drugstore)
into a pillowcase the same color as the bed linen or the chair on
which the patient sits. Thus you protect bedding, and are cam-
ouflaging the patient's need for extra absorbency.

• After an incontinent episode immediately wash the patient
and then dry thoroughly. Ask your patient to do this himself
whenever possible.

• Ask the physician or nurse for additional ways to care for
your patient's condition.

• Consider the Dignity approach to incontinence. These are
knit underpants with replaceable high-absorbency pads; their appearance is relatively innocuous. For information write: Human-
icare International Inc., 5 Joanna Court, East Brunswick, N.J.
08816.

What About Catheter Care?

A catheter is a narrow tube inserted through the urethra into
the bladder. It allows urine to flow outside the body. Most are
inserted by a physician or nurse. Some care givers are asked to
insert catheters, but it is the exception, not the rule. If you are
required to insert a catheter you will be given explicit instructions
and supervision by a medical professional.

Catheter Troubleshooting
Does your patient have a catheter? Then, be sure to:
• keep the urinary meatus (opening into the bladder) clean.
Wash that area and perineal area between anus and genitals during
bath or shower.
• watch for discharge. In women vaginal discharge can con-
taminate the catheter. In men, watch for bleeding through the

penis which can be caused by urinary tract infections or irritation from the catheter.

• keep catheter clean with soap and water. Be sure it is dry after washing.

• never elevate the collection bag and risk return flow of urine into the bladder.

Enemas

Certainly, giving an enema is one of the most inelegant of all home-care tasks. Enemas are intended to relieve the distress of constipation or prepare a person for a diagnostic test. Commercial preparations are inexpensive, fast, and nearly effortless. Or you may be told to use an enema bag and add a specially mixed liquid prescribed by the physician.

Get explicit instructions from the nurse or doctor. Then do the following.

1. Try to relax your patient as this will make things easier. Also be sure that any water used for the enema is comfortably warm, not hot. Position your patient on his/her left side in a knee to chest position. This will enable the enema solution to flow into intestines and make the laxative effective.

2. Lubricate the enema's tube with Vaseline, K-Y Jelly, or mineral oil for comfortable insertion.

3. Let the patient know what you intend to do. Then insert the tube about four inches—less in young children. Allow liquid to flow into the patient.

4. Ask the patient to hold the liquid as long as directions indicate (usually about twenty minutes, but check with physician). If your patient has trouble with this, ask him/her to try for the best. For the bedridden, have a bedpan or commode nearby in case your patient needs to eliminate suddenly. For ambulatory patients, allow the patient to sit on the toilet while holding the enema liquid. The extra security of the toilet may enable the patient to hold the liquid longer.

5. After the liquid has been held for the prescribed time, ask the patient to release contents into toilet or bedpan.

Home-Care Basic #10: Giving Medication

Chances are you may find administering medication to your patient a bit confusing. It's a problem that I faced—tackled and beat. Let me show you the way.

There's no substitute for being totally informed about the medication your patient must take. In this way you can spot side effects and ineffectiveness, and know when to call the physician about problems. My advice:

• Know the medication's name. Most go by trade rather than generic names. For example, the trade name Valium is more familiar than its generic equivalent, diazepam. Tip: Ask physician to prescribe generic drugs whenever possible—they're cheaper.

• Know the drug's use and possible side effects. Check out the *United States Pharmacopeia/Dispensing Information (USP/ DI)*—a big name for a fabulous reference. Here, in simple language, you will learn all you need to know about prescribed drugs. Another source is the *Physician's Desk Reference*. A new one is published each year (as is the *USP/DI*). But the *PDR* may be a bit technical for some lay people. Both are at your library.

• Know the answers to these questions: How often should the drug be taken? How many days should the drug be taken? Are there special instructions (take with meals, juice, before bed, etc.)? What are the patient's known allergies? Will the drug react with others the patient takes? What side effects may occur? When should you call the physician about the medication? If the drug must be taken for a long time, what are the long-term effects? Some can damage certain organs. Is your patient pregnant? If so, know that certain drugs have a negative effect on the growing fetus and may affect succeeding generations. (This includes self-medication with drugs purchased without prescription.)

Sorting Out the Most Effective Ways to Give Medicine

• capsules: Difficulty swallowing? Pour contents into juice or applesauce. Warning: Don't remove medication from capsules without physician's approval. This can alter the effects of some drugs. With time-release capsules, each dot of medication inside the capsule dissolves at a different rate inside the body. Never empty these capsules into food or liquid. This interferes with the time-release benefit of the drug and the patient can receive an accidental overdose.

• liquids: Unpleasant taste? Make them more palatable by mixing in applesauce, juice, or flavored syrup. Use caution, however, when doing this with children. Associations of medications with certain foods can turn the child off to that food. Tip: To avoid spills use a medicine cup instead of a spoon or, use a Super Dropper. It holds a full medically defined teaspoon as it delivers medication in the back of the mouth, behind the taste buds. Buy at drugstore or write Apex Medical Supply, Inc., P.O. Box 20171, Bloomington, Minn. 55420 for catalogue.

• suppositories: For sanitary insertion use rubber finger cots. (They cover fingertips and are disposable.) Purchase at drugstore, surgical supply.

• tablets: Swallowing difficulties? Ask the physician if the drug comes in liquid or powder form. Some can be crushed. Some cannot as this can alter the drug's effect. Ask physician or pharmacist for guidance.

• powders: If you must apply to skin or wound, don't use bare fingertips. Sprinkle required amount on a sterile gauze pad. Then dab affected area.

• troches: These medications are designed to alleviate discomfort in the mouth and throat as they dissolve. Tell your patient not to chew troches. Why? Because slow dissolving brings a higher concentration of the drug to the affected area.

What Do You Do When You Accidentally Skip a Dose?

Don't panic. In most cases one skipped dose is not a problem. However, you shouldn't double the next dose to compensate. Call the physician for instructions.

How to Give a Reluctant Child Medication— and Save Your Sanity

So many mothers are exasperated by this problem. My suggestion is to relax your child by appearing relaxed yourself. I know how tempting it is to want to raise your voice. Instead, try to project calm—it's contagious. And it's likely that if you administer medication to your child in a matter-of-fact way your little one will eventually cooperate. If, however, difficulty persists, call the pediatrician and ask for advice. Sometimes a medicine dose can be skipped. Occasionally some medications must be given by injection.

Two more things to remember are (1) encourage your child's trust by being honest. Never say that a medicine will taste good when it won't. Your child won't believe you next time. Try asking the physician if the medicine can be prescribed in another, more palatable form. And (2) don't treat medicine like candy. Your little one may be tempted to look for the "candy" later and risk an accidental overdose.

And When an Adult Refuses Medication?

To be sure, this is everyone's right. Perhaps the experience of a visiting nurse I met can help you solve this problem. When her patient refused medication the nurse asked, "Why don't you want it? Does it taste bad? Does it cause side effects?" She reminded the patient that these were legitimate reasons. The patient said that after each dose he felt nauseated. The nurse called the physician and the medication was changed. The solution is often that simple.

For other patients, noncompliance may be a way to control a recovery situation where everything is being done for them. Your patient may be sending you messages that he or she is annoyed, depressed, upset, or frightened. Provoke conversation to get to the bottom of your loved one's feelings. If you create an atmosphere of interest and support, you may find that your patient will open up and honestly speak his or her mind.

Tips for Giving Medication to Confused and Disoriented Patients

Semiconscious, disoriented, senile, or confused patients need special attention when it comes to medication. Always administer it yourself. Be sure patient is sitting upright. Never allow this patient to take medication on his or her own. Stand by to watch if the drug works or if it causes side effects. Are you nervous about giving medication to this type of person? Are you worried that he or she will choke or gag? In most cases the individual's gag reflex works to keep such accidents from happening. However, for additional peace of mind, read the life-saving techniques for choking victims in Chapter 10.

Your Miniguide to Radiation and Chemotherapy

What Is Radiation Therapy?

It's the use of high-energy rays to halt the growing and multiplying of cancer cells. If your patient has had this treatment he or she may have had external radiation therapy (a machine aims high-energy rays on the cancer) or internal radiation therapy (tiny pieces of radioactive material are implanted directly on the cancer and left for a brief time).

What Are the Side Effects?

Not all radiation therapy patients experience side effects. However, if side effects do develop they usually occur when the patient is well into treatments. Tell the physician about any side effects your patient suffers. You should know that these effects may last for a few weeks after therapy is completed. They include fatigue, appetite loss, skin irritations, stomach or abdominal distress and diarrhea. Radiation to the lungs can cause coughing and shortness of breath; to the head, hair loss; to the abdomen or groin area, sterility and birth defects.

How Can You Ease Your Patient's Discomfort?

I have included many suggestions in Chapter 6 to help you restore lost appetites. Your goal should be to help maintain your patient's strength and normal weight during this time so that he or she can fight illness and cope with the treatments.

Rest and good nutrition can help beat fatigue. Furthermore, you can contact your local American Cancer Society or Cancer Information Service. They have information about publications and services designed to make a cancer patient's life more pleasant.

Skin effects such as irritation, tanning, or sunburn, are temporary and will clear up when treatments are finished. Just don't aggravate the condition by putting something warm against your patient's sensitive skin (a hot water or heating pad, for example). And don't apply perfumes, ointments, or cosmetics to the irritated area.

Radiation treatment to the stomach or abdominal area frequently can cause upset stomach and diarrhea. Clear liquid diets are often helpful at these times—especially during bouts of nausea and diarrhea. Have your patient drink lots of liquids to replace the ones that are lost. Tip: Avoid milk and milk products as they tend to make diarrhea worse.

What Is Chemotherapy?

Here, anticancer drugs are given orally, by injection, or intravenously. These drugs travel throughout the body to reach and destroy cancer cells. Unfortunately, chemotherapy can affect normal cells too, such as bone marrow, gastrointestinal tract, reproductive system, and hair follicles.

It's worth noting here that the side effects that your patient feels have little to do with the drug's effectiveness. The potency of the drug to kill cancer cells is not measured by the intensity or amount of side effects your loved one may have. Some individuals receive effective treatment without any side effects.

How Can You Ease Your Patient's Discomfort?

Again, see Chapter 6 for information about lifting sagging appetites and providing your patient with good nutrition.

Your patient is particularly susceptible to illness at this time because chemotherapy reduces the body's ability to fight infection. How? By affecting the bone marrow that produces germ-fighting white cells. So keep your patient away from people who have contagious diseases such as flu, measles, chicken pox. *Watch out for these warning signs of infection*: temperature over 100°F, diarrhea for forty-eight hours, cough, burning sensation when urinating, chills, sore throat. Call physician immediately if you observe any of these signs.

If your patient has blood clotting problems, it is important to avoid injury. Avoid giving aspirin at this time because it may cause the chemotherapy patient to bleed more easily. Watch out for easy bruising or red spots under the skin. Also, check for bleeding from potential trouble spots such as gums, nose, or in urine and bowel movements. Call the physician immediately if any of these danger signs appear.

Hair loss may be a disturbing sign for your patient. It is a temporary side effect, yet it can be traumatic. Naturally, you may want to consider hairpieces, scarfs, hats, and so forth. My advice: If you know that your patient needs chemotherapy, try to make arrangements for wigs or hair pieces *before* treatment. Once therapy starts your patient may not feel well enough to deal with such purchases.

Other side effects such as muscle weakness, skin dryness, and itching should be discussed with the physician for more detailed care instructions.

Some chemotherapy drugs may cause changes in urine color. For example, Adriamycin may cause it to turn red. Methotrexate can turn it bright yellow.

Finally, chemotherapy can affect a person's reproductive system. Not only do these drugs have the ability to damage the unborn fetus, but, in men, chemotherapy often causes a decrease in sperm production which can affect male fertility. Discuss with the physician the possibility of having sperm frozen to allow for artificial insemination if desired at a future time.

How to Give Medication When Your Patient Feels Nauseated

Did you know that some medications come in suppository forms? If your patient has difficulty swallowing, this method can be a handy way to retain each medicine dose.

Also, the doctor may be able to prescribe an antiemetic (antinausea) drug for the nauseated patient to take before food or medication.

Perhaps the medication your patient is taking is causing the nausea or vomiting. Consult the physician immediately if you suspect this. On the other hand, some drugs cause nausea when taken on an empty stomach, so follow specific instructions for taking these substances with food when indicated.

What should you do if your patient vomits after taking medication? Obviously he or she has lost a dose of something that may be needed for recovery. Call the physician and ask if the medicine should be repeated.

The Panic-Proof Way to Organize and Administer Medication

One of the areas of home care that caused me the most anxiety was juggling my father's many medications and trying to remember to follow the specific instructions for each. At one time I dealt with six different pills. Each had to be given at a different hour. One had side effects that had to be monitored. Another was to be given only if certain side effects occurred. Every time I had to face this medicine maze I panicked. Then I stumbled on a solution: the Medication Sheet and the Pill Organizer.

I made up the Medication Sheet to list all the drugs I had to administer (see Chapter 2). I included the drug's name, dose, special directions, and possible side effects, and tacked it onto the box that held all medications (use a shoe box, cigar box, etc. You may want to tack the sheet on the refrigerator door or by your patient's bedside.) Whenever I administered a drug, I checked off the appropriate box (see Figure 2). In addition, I used a Pill Organizer.

The Pill Organizer is a device you can buy at the drug store. It is a plastic case that has compartments labeled for each day of the week. At the start of the week (or illness) fill each compartment with the appropriate pills. By the end of the day your patient should have received all the medication in the specific compartment. (A small slip of paper in each compartment can serve as a reminder to administer liquids and other drugs inappropriate for the Pill Organizer.) Make your own organizer by using an old egg box or tackle box, or taping together seven paper cups. Be sure containers are tightly covered—too much exposure to air can make some medications ineffective. Keep this and all other medications away from children.

Perhaps your patient doesn't take pills, but is taking a variety of liquids, ointments, and so on. In such cases the Medication Sheet by itself should do the trick.

Drug Interaction Do's and Don'ts

Some things can interact with medication to produce a negative effect on the body. Be on the lookout for these risky combos.

• drugs and alcohol: Don't combine alcohol with sedatives, hypnotics, barbiturates, central nervous system depressants, antihistamines and tranquilizers. Check with pharmacist to find out if alcohol should not be taken with the medication prescribed.

• drugs and water: Some need lots of water to work properly. Give your patient plenty of water when he or she is taking sulfa drugs such as Bactrim, Septra, Zyloprim (allopurinol), Metamucil, aspirin.

• aspirin and anticoagulants: Don't take anticoagulants with aspirin. Also called blood thinners, these drugs can cause serious internal bleeding if taken in combination with aspirin. Moreover, any new drugs taken with anticoagulants must be checked with the physician.

• mineral oil and vitamins: If your patient is taking multivitamins don't give him or her mineral oil—it can diminish the vitamin's effectiveness.

• antacids: They can destroy the effect of drugs with enteric coatings.

• MAO Inhibitors: These drugs can be fatal if ingested with these foods: cheese, pickled herring, and wine and certain other medications. (See Chapter 11 for additional list.)

• diuretics and steroids: Both can cause potassium depletion, which can lead to serious health problems. Patients taking these drugs should be eating potassium rich diets including foods such as bananas, orange juice, dried fruits (raisins, apricots, etc.), prune juice.

• drugs and the sun: Some medications can increase a person's sensitivity to sunlight. Tetracycline is the most common offender. Consult the physician to see if any of your patient's drugs may have a similar effect.

Home-Care Basic #11:
Home Care After Heart Attack

Your patient is home after a heart attack. No doubt his or her medical needs have been taken care of, and now your loved one is faced with the emotional and physical adjustments of recovery. You will both benefit if you have a deeper understanding of what your patient is going through.

A heart attack is the result of a slow and progressive condition called atherosclerosis. The arteries that supply the heart with blood are narrowed by cholesterol (fat) deposits. In time this can create a blockage making it impossible for blood to flow to the heart. This condition takes years to develop and it's possible that your patient did not have any warning signs. When the attack occurs a small part of the heart "dies" because the essential supply of oxygen-carrying blood is unable to reach it. Stress and hered- itary factors are also believed to be significant contributors to coronary artery disease.

It's likely that now your patient is home you are feeling fearful, worried, even guilty. Do you think that you "gave" your patient a heart attack? Nonsense. There are specific physical reasons for heart attacks over which you have no control. If you are over- whelmed by fears or guilt, it's best to talk over these emotions with a physician, nurse, or psychologist.

As for your patient, he or she is encountering a constellation of feelings. Fear is common. "Am I living on borrowed time?" many patients ask. Every chest pain may trigger the fear tha another attack is imminent. "It's *your* fault," may be a messag that you pick up. It's not your fault, so don't fall into that gui trap. Probably the most common complaint is that the patien does not feel like a whole person. You may hear, "I'm not the same as I used to be," or "I'm an old man/woman." What should you do? Be patient and accepting. In most cases these fears fade away. Most patients survive their first attacks and go on to resume normal lives. Naturally, many activities must be curtailed at first, such as exercise, work, and sex. Check with the physician to learn exactly what your patient can and cannot do. Most often physicians advise their patients to rest while the heart heals, then to resume normal activities slowly, usually in six to eight weeks. Diet changes and weight reduction may also be prescribed for your patient. For additional information about heart attacks and special diets, contact your local Heart Association.

What About Chest Pains?

There are pains that may signal a heart attack and those that announce *angina*. Angina is a condition where the heart muscle doesn't get enough blood. This causes chest pain often felt in the left arm and shoulder. It is a temporary pain that's often alleviated with a drug called nitroglycerine.

How to Tell When an Angina Patient Is Having a Heart Attack

Get emergency help if your angina patient has an *obvious change in the pattern of pain* such as:
• the pain feels "different" or there is a new distribution of pain—for example, the new pain may radiate
• the pain occurs more often than usual
• the pain is not helped by prescribed medication
• the pain occurs at unusual times—for example, at rest, while sleeping, etc.
• severe pain, dizziness, fainting, sweating, nausea, or shortness of breath accompany chest pain.

Important: Many heart-attack victims die needlessly because they don't get medical help fast enough. True, not all deaths can be prevented. But you may be able to save a loved one's life if you recognize the warning signs and act quickly. One of the most dangerous time-wasters is the patient who denies what's happening. Take prompt action at the slightest possibility of an attack. It only takes *one* warning sign to warrant a trip to the hospital emergency room (see Chapter 10).

Home-Care Basic #12: Assistive Devices to Make Your Patient's Life Easier

Wheelchair Savvy

This is an expensive piece of equipment that I advise you to buy with care. I suggest that you get a physician's prescription and a referral to an occupational therapist. The therapist is trained to fit your patient with the chair that's most suited to his or her life-style. Don't buy a chair without the advice of a medical professional. You may buy the wrong type and waste good money. One therapist told me about a husband who bought a wheelchair for his wife on his own. The chair was not adjusted properly to her size; nor was it designed to negotiate their home's narrow hallways or slide underneath tabletops. An occupational therapist would have ordered a chair to make the woman's life easier— not more difficult.

Your patient may choose from these types of chairs:

• standard: The basic wheelchair with immovable armrests. Most often this chair must be fitted with special features to adapt to a patient's special needs.

• amputee wheelchair: This is specially designed to compensate for the weight of lost limbs.

• recliner wheelchair: This unit is intended for people with very limited head and trunk support.

• hemiplegic chair: Designed for individuals who are paralyzed on one side.

• large wheelchairs: The standard size chair built bigger to accommodate large patients.

• narrow wheelchairs: These models save space and enable the patient to manage narrow aisles and doorways.

All the above chairs can be fitted with a host of special features. Here's a small sampling: seat cushions to reduce risk of pressure sores; movable arms to allow sliding to and from the chair to the bed, toilet, car, etc.; commode seats and pans to allow the chair to convert into a toilet.

The Electric Wheelchair: When Is It the Right Choice?

When the choice is made in collaboration with an occupational therapist. Indeed, these chairs are not for all disabled patients. They are difficult to regulate unless the individual has use of at least one hand. They are difficult to get up and down curbs (often impossible). They are heavy, sometimes needing two strong people to lift them. They are not always practical at home because they may be troublesome when negotiating tight spaces, furniture, and carpeting. They are often difficult to move manually if the motor breaks down.

However, when fitted to the right patient they can be a godsend—enabling the person to travel longer distances without the wear and tear of the standard chair and allowing greater independence.

The latest alternative to the standard electric wheelchair is the modified scooter. This is a motorized chair that looks like a scooter with a narrower construction and similar steering mechanisms. I mention this wonderful device because it has several strong pluses over the conventional models. It doesn't look medical, which can boost a patient's self-esteem. It has a narrow turning radius, which makes it easier to steer than conventional models. It can get through narrow doorways and aisles. It is easier to disassemble and to get in and out of a car than standard chairs.

Where to Buy or Rent Wheelchairs

I recommend that you ask the occupational therapist for guidance here. Two companies known to supply top-quality conventional vehicles are Everest & Jennings, Inc., 3233 Mission Oaks Blvd., Camarillo, Calif. 93010 and Invacare, P.O. Box 4028, Elyria, Ohio 44036. Write for their free catalogues. Or contact a surgical supply store.

As for the modified scooter seats, a reliable machine used with much success is manufactured by the AMIGO company. Write for a free catalogue to AMIGO Sales, Inc., 6693 Dixie Hwy., Bridgeport, Mich. 48722.

Wheelchair Care

Every chair comes equipped with an owner's manual with specific instructions for lubrication and maintenance. Here are some general highlights to remember.

• metal parts: Wipe with soft cloth once a week. Use chrome polish once a month.

• upholstery: Repair small tears with tape to lessen tearing. Apply a Naugahyde conditioner once a month.

• tires: See manual for specific care instructions.

For indoor use you will find it necessary to arrange furniture so that the chair can be maneuvered easily in and out of rooms. A low-pile carpeting will not snag wheels and makes movement easier.

How to Transfer Your Patient to and from the Wheelchair

It is important that you get supervised instructions from a physical or occupational therapist. He or she will show you proper body mechanics so that you can avoid injury to yourself or the patient during transfers. To supplement their instructions:

1. The chair must not move during transfer. Lock wheels. Prepare your body before transfer by standing close to the patient. (The farther away you stand the greater the strain on your back.) Keep feet apart, one foot ahead of the other to give yourself support and balance. (Legs kept together interfere with proper balance and can lead to falling with the patient.)

2. Maintain a straight back, but keep hips and knees bent. Straighten your legs as you assist the patient into a standing position.

3. Be sure your patient can see the surface to which he/she is transferring. Don't block his/her vision.

4. If the patient is wearing a catheter to catch urine, don't pull the catheter during transfer. This could injure the patient.

Crutches

Standard axillary crutches are made of wood with rubber tips at the bottom. To get the safest and most efficient use from them your patient must be fitted by a professional therapist or nurse. Once they've been adjusted it's important that the patient does not bear weight on the underarm (axillary) cross bar. Why? Because that can impair the nerves or arteries that supply the arm and hand. Called "crutch palsy," the early warning signs are weakness or numbness of the arm. Once it occurs it can make crutch use difficult, sometimes impossible.

Self-Help Aids to Make Your Patient More Independent

If your patient has a long-term illness or disability you will be interested to know that there are many commercially made devices to make both your lives easier. These include:

bed boards	pressure-sore preventors
oxygen units	cast protectors
hydraulic patient lifters	wheelchairs and accessories
tapes, bandages, dressings	in-bed shampoo trays
walking aids	blood pressure equipment
eating aids	post-mastectomy products
ostomy products	bath and shower safety devices
raised toilet seats	incontinent-care equipment

You may also want to consult a physician or nurse, although an occupational therapist is probably your best bet for advice about self-help aids.

Another solution is to browse through mail-order catalogues that list and describe home-care equipment. In this way you can learn what's available. Then, if you wish, you can order by mail through your local surgical or medical supply dealer or with the help of an occupational therapist.

Check out these companies and their catalogues for a wide variety of choices.

• Maddak Inc. (Pequannock, N.J. 07440) publishes a catalogue that displays self-help aids and home health-care equipment. They manufacture many of their own products which are available through surgical supply dealers around the country.

• Fred Sammons, Inc. (Box 32, Brookfield, Ill. 60513) has been in the business of supplying self-help aids to professionals for twenty-five years. Ask your local surgical supply dealer or occupational therapist about Sammons' product line, which includes eating, dressing, wheelchair, recreation, and communication aids.

• Sola Designs, Inc., Selected Objects for Living Actively (242 West 27th St., New York, N.Y. 10001) designs objects for people with disabilities. They are unique because they are not just functional—they're beautiful. Their catalogue lists utensils for eating, special dishes, and furniture. Order directly from Sola.

• Kagle Home-Health Services (4422 Bronx Blvd., Bronx, N.Y. 10470) publishes an illustrated catalogue of in-home health products. Order directly from Kagle.

• The National Easter Seal Society, Information Service (2023 West Ogden Ave., Chicago, Ill. 60612) helps provide equipment needed by individuals recovering from either short- or long-term disabilities. Equipment is available for loan or purchase and includes wheelchairs, geriatric chairs, walkers, hospital beds, bed rails, trapeze bars, patient lifters, bathtub grab bars, canes, and crutches. For more information about equipment and home-care publications contact your local Easter Seal Society or write to above address.

• Edmund Scientific for Health and Fitness (101 E. Gloucester Pike, Barrington, N.J. 08007) offers a catalogue with a varied selection of self-health aids such as blood-pressure equipment, first-aid kits, biofeedback machines. Order directly from Edmund Scientific.

• The Whitaker Company (41 Douglas Ave., Yonkers, N.Y. 10703) specializes in lifting devices to help disabled persons. Their products include seat-lift chairs, wheelchair lifts, bath lifts, electric wheelchairs. Ask for catalogue.

• Inclinator Company of America (2200 Paxton St., P.O. Box 1557, Harrisburg, Pa. 17105) issues a brochure that pictures in-home elevators, stair lifts, and custom-built dumbwaiters.

• J. T. Posey Company (5635 Peck Rd., Arcadia, Calif. 91006) supplies many home-care aids including foot-guards and other items to protect against pressure sores.

• FashionAble (P.O. Box S, Rocky Hill, N.J. 08553) offers a catalogue called *Self-Help Items for Independent Living*. Know that in addition to a variety of assistive devices, FashionAble specializes in easy-on, easy-off clothing.

• St. Louis Ostomy & Medical Supply, Inc. (10821 Man-chester Rd., St. Louis, Mo. 63122) supplies free literature about urinary supplies, assistive devices, ostomy products, and reha-bilitation equipment.

• Urocare Products, Inc. (2419 Merced Ave., South El Monte, Calif. 91733) specializes in products for incontinent patients. Send for illustrated catalogue.

• Comfortably Yours (52 West Hunter Ave., Maywood, N.J. 07607) offers unique products to enhance comfort for the ill or disabled.

In addition, you may want to consider these two publications: *Aids to Make You Able*, by Wendy M. Davis, Beaufort Books, Inc. New York (includes tips on assistive devices to make life easier for disabled persons, suggestions for improving equipment as well as buying it; $8.95); and *Source Book for the Disabled*, edited by Gloria Hale, Bantam Books, New York (a listing of resources for disabled people—adults and children—and instruc-tions for adapting the home to assistive devices; $3.95).

Home-Care Basic #13:
You *Can* Beat Cabin Fever and Boredom!

Cabin fever. You've had a taste of it if you've ever been cooped up at home for a few days or more with a cold or the flu. You know the signs: isolation, loneliness, boredom.

Long-term home-care patients may suffer severe cases of "cabin fever." And that can lead to irritability and a profound depression. Prevent this unpleasantness by providing distracting and pleasurable activities for your patient.

Start by asking yourself what your loved one's favorite sources of entertainment and pleasure were before illness. Now try to discover, with the help of a medical professional, which activities are medically possible in the home setting. Here are some suggestions for activities that have worked for others.

For adults:

reading (large print publications for visually impaired)

being read to

knitting, sewing, crocheting

letter writing

card games

board games

plant care

start an herb garden

carpentry work

home computers

drawing, painting

television, radio

video games

video cassettes

telephone calls

music/radio listening

baking

For children, many of the above activities in addition to:

playing make-believe with toy characters

stamp/coin/shell collecting

model building

dressing up in costume

whittling

sewing

doll making

singing songs

crafts using clay, paper, glue, wood, fabric

making a scrapbook from magazine pictures

How to Use Music to Bring Joy to Your Loved One

A friend of mine cared for her terminally ill father at home. She wanted to make his days calm and comfortable.

After a while she discovered that music was a miraculous tranquilizer, spirit lifter and entertainer. Her bedridden father spent hours enjoying nostalgic melodies, rich harmonies, and diverting vocalists.

You, too, can use music to take the edge off your patient's isolation. Find out his or her favorite style of music, or experiment on your own. This may be done inexpensively by borrowing records from friends, neighbors, or the library.

Use music to set a mood. For example, to relax your patient play tunes with simple harmonies, slow tempos, and few dynamic changes. Try gentle instrumentals and mellow classical music.

To stimulate activity, select pieces with lots of abrupt tempo changes. Drums and other percussion instruments can supply invigorating sounds.

Moreover, you can entertain a child or adult by playing records or tapes that are rich with words. Broadway show tunes and comedy records are examples.

Pick old favorites. Such music often inspires memories that can fire conversations as you and your patient reminisce about times past.

One more thing: Music doesn't have to be a passive experience. Your patient can participate in it, too. For instance, he or she can play an instrument or take music lessons at home. Or perhaps you can start a sing-a-long involving the whole family. Not only can this be an uplifting experience, it can also make your loved one feel part of things.

Companionship: People and Pets

People give life. Patients who are alone much of the time are deprived of the healing powers of human warmth and companionship. Indeed, loneliness can fill a person with pain far more searing than physical distress.

Not all home-care patients live with families. Many, especially the elderly, are on their own. If you have a relative or friend who is in this situation, I strongly urge you to try to change it. When family, friends, or neighbors are unavailable for visits, turn to paid companions or volunteers.

Part-time or live-in companions may be located by contacting your local visiting nurses association. Or check in the Yellow Pages under "Home-Care Services" or "Nurses." You will see agencies that supply companions. Regarding volunteers, churches and synagogues are excellent sources. Contact a social worker, county social services department, or Yellow Pages to learn more about volunteer organizations in your patient's community.

As for pets, don't sell short their powers. Recent research shows that for people living alone pets have sparked remarkable transformations enabling severely disabled people to cope better with their disabilities and helping depressed individuals to become more socially active.

Along these lines, you've probably heard of Seeing Eye dogs for the blind. But did you know that there are "hearing ear" dogs for the deaf? And dogs that can be trained to fetch and retrieve for and assist people who are bedridden or wheelchair-bound?

Research is being done in this field around the country. For more information about the therapeutic uses of animals contact the University of Pennsylvania School of Veterinary Medicine, Center for the Interaction of Animals and Society, 3800 Spruce St., Philadelphia, Pa. 19104.

4

Nursing Skills to Turn You into the Doctor's Care-Partner

Would you know what to do if the physician asked you to take your patient's *vital signs*? That's the temperature, pulse, respiration, or blood pressure.

Readings from the vitals provide the clues that medical professionals need to assess a person's condition. They signal changes in health and warn of medical emergencies. In short, they are nursing skills you shouldn't be without.

On the following pages I will show you how to take each sign, how to record results, and which readings mean trouble. Let me add that these pages are not intended to encourage you to make diagnoses. That's your physician's job. Use these skills to *assist* your physician, not replace him or her.

Vital Sign #1: Temperature

When temperature rises above the patient's average normal range, it is called fever. Normal is between 97.2°F. and 99.5°F. orally. Rectal temperature may normally reach 100.5°F.

Fever may be caused by many things, including infection, drug reactions, certain cancer treatments, some types of arthritis, and so on.

What you probably don't know is that fever by itself does not tell a physician a whole lot. Expect him or her to ask you questions about other health clues that may shed light on your patient's condition. These include rash, pain, prolonged fever, chills, confusion, vomiting, loss of appetite, weakness, nausea, sweating, convulsions, restlessness, headache.

Fever Alert

> 100°F.—mild fever
> 102°F.—moderate fever
> 103°F. and above—call physician to find out how to lower fever. Do not automatically use aspirin to reduce fever (especially high fever) in children. Also there is some evidence that aspirin used to fight fevers in children with flu or chicken pox can lead to other health complications. Ask the pediatrician for advice.

• Notify physician at once if a child under two develops a fever higher than 102°F. Febrile convulsions can occur when there is high fever in certain susceptible children. Institute temperature lowering procedures when fever rises above 102°F. (see Chapter 8). If there is no change, call physician as soon as possible.

• Notify physician immediately if fever occurs after institution of a new medication or treatment. Some drugs, for example, have a fever-inducing side effect in susceptible persons. The list is long. The most common are antihistamines, aspirin (yes! in some people), Aldomet, barbiturates, Dilantin, sulfa drugs, penicillin, quinidine.

• Know if your patient's condition can cause fever. For instance, some people with diabetes, congestive heart failure, or cancer may experience fever as a result of their illness.

How to Bring Down a High Fever

• Call the physician for exact instructions. Note the controversy about aspirin and high fevers in children (see Chapter 8) as indicated above. Do not administer aspirin to a child with a high fever unless you receive the okay from the pediatrician.

• One way to lower fever without medication is to immerse the patient in cool or lukewarm water below his or her recorded body temperature. For example, if your patient has a 103°F. fever the water should be between 98°F. and 100°F. A bathtub thermometer can help you get the most accurate readings. However, before any attempt to reduce a fever is made, call physician for guidance.

How to Take Oral Temperature

Here you use an *oral thermometer*. It is placed in the mouth under the tongue and is not advisable for infants, young children, paralyzed individuals, confused patients and after oral surgery. Purchase the thermometer at the drugstore or surgical supply store. Recognize it by its long, slender bulb. Cost: about $2.

1. Check thermometer before using. Be sure numbers and lines are readable, and that the glass tube is not cracked or broken.

2. Disinfect thermometer by dipping it in rubbing alcohol. Rinse off with cool water. If thermometer is being used repeatedly for the same person, soap and water will do after each use. Never wash it in hot water—it will break.

3. Shake down thermometer before taking temperature, holding the end opposite the silver bulb. Use a strong flick-of-the-wrist action to shake down the mercury. Get a reading below 95°F. (usually takes three vigorous shakes).

4. Be sure patient has not chewed gum, just eaten, brushed teeth, smoked, or drunk anything hot or cold before taking oral temperature, as accurate readings can be altered in each instance.

5. Insert thermometer, bulb first, into the mouth and under the tongue as far back as possible. Ask patient to close lips tightly

around thermometer—not to bite, chew, or dislodge it. Warning: *Never leave children or confused patients alone with an oral thermometer in their mouths.*

6. Ask patient to sit as still as possible for three minutes, then remove thermometer.

7. To read the thermometer, hold it up to the light. Read mercury column, which appears as a silver streak, where it falls between the lines and numbers on the glass tube. It may be necessary to turn the tube slowly until it catches light. Read the long line to the left where the mercury column has stopped. This will be a full degree (92, 93, 94, etc.). Write this number on the

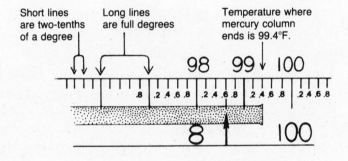

Figure 5. How to Read a Thermometer

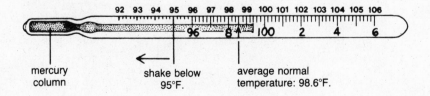

Home-Health Chart. Then count the short lines to the right until the mercury stops. Each line equals two-tenths of a point (.2, .4, .6, etc.). The two numbers combined equal the oral temperature. (See Figure 5.)

8. When finished, clean the thermometer with rubbing alcohol and put it in a safe place away from children.

What if the Thermometer Breaks Inside the Mouth?

• Tell the patient not to swallow.

• Tell patient to spit out all contents immediately.

• If patient has swallowed glass have him/her eat bread and call physician immediately.

• If you have *any* doubt as to whether or not the patient swallowed glass call physician. Mercury alone in this form is usually harmless.

How to Take Rectal Temperature

Use a *rectal thermometer*. It is placed inside the anus and is not advisable for patients who have had recent surgery on or near the area of the rectum. It is commonly used on children under six, confused persons, paralyzed patients, patients with breathing difficulties and oral surgery patients. Purchase thermometer at the drugstore or surgical supply store. Recognize it by its short bulb. Cost: about $2.

1. Check thermometer before using. Be sure the numbers and lines are readable, and that the glass tube is not cracked or broken.

2. Disinfect the thermometer by dipping it in rubbing alcohol and rinsing it off with water. Never wash the thermometer in hot water; it will break.

3. Shake down thermometer before taking temperature. Before inserting into patient's anus, hold the end opposite the silver bulb. Use a strong flick of the wrist to bring down the mercury in the glass tube. Shake below 95°F.; usually takes three vigorous shakes.

4. Allow patient as much privacy as needed.

5. Position patient in comfortable side-lying or supine position with one leg flexed.

6. Remove clothing from around anus; uncover smallest area necessary for insertion.

7. Lubricate thermometer bulb and lowest portion of thermometer. (Possible lubricants: Vaseline, cold cream, sterile lubricating jelly, soap).

8. Insert thermometer about one and a half inches for adults, less for children. Keep in place for two to three minutes.

9. Ask patient not to roll over or move while thermometer is in place.

10. If patient is an infant or child or confused or unconscious, hold the thermometer in place to prevent dislodging. Instructions for young children: Place a very young child down on the bed or hold across your knees. Hold child's buttocks in the palm of your hand allowing the thermometer to poke out between the second and third fingers. Keep thermometer in place for about three to five minutes. (See Figure 6.)

Figure 6. Temperature Taking for Young Child

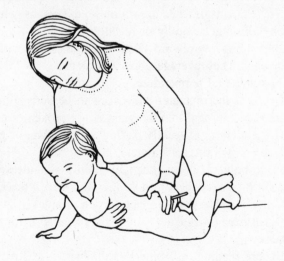

11. Rectal temperatures average one degree higher than oral. To read temperature hold thermometer up to the light. Read mercury column where it falls between lines and numbers on the glass tube. It may be necessary to turn the tube slowly until it catches the light. Read the long line to the left where the mercury column has stopped. This is a full degree (92, 93, 94, etc.). Write this number on the Home-Health Chart. Then count the short lines to the right until the mercury stops. Each line equals two-tenths of a point (.2, .4, .6, etc.). The two numbers combined equal the temperature.

12. When finished, clean the thermometer with rubbing alcohol and put it in a safe place away from children.

What if the Thermometer Breaks Inside the Rectum?

Do not try to remove it. Such efforts may push the glass tube and/or contents deeper into the patient. Ask patient to stay on stomach and call physician immediately for guidance.

How to Take Axillary Temperature

This method is used when oral and rectal temperatures cannot be taken. Patients include newborns and persons who cannot accept a thermometer orally or rectally.

Axillary temperatures are taken under the arm with an oral thermometer. They average about one degree less than the patient's average oral temperature.

1. Use oral thermometer and check to be sure numbers and lines are readable, and that the glass is not broken or cracked.

2. Dry underarm by gently patting with a towel or gauze.

3. Shake down the thermometer below 95°F.

4. Place bulb of thermometer in middle of underarm. Place patient's arm across chest to hold thermometer in place.

5. Leave thermometer in place for ten minutes.

6. Read thermometer the same way you read it for oral temperature.

7. Record reading on Home-Health Chart.

How to Record Temperature Readings

No matter how simple or elaborate your patient's chart, be sure to include this information each time you take the temperature: temperature reading, time, and method.

Vital Sign #2: Pulse

Pulse is the perceptible expansion and contraction of an artery when felt by the fingers. It tells medical professionals the power, rate, and rhythm of the heartbeat. Pulse can be felt at various spots on the body called *pulse points*.

Your patient's pulse may fluctuate more dramatically than any of the other vital signs. The reason: It's affected by many things such as excitement, anxiety, sleep, medication, temperature, and exertion. Pulse provides clues to a person's underlying condition—from the presence of infection to impending medical emergencies.

An isolated change in pulse may not mean much unless it occurs with other signs. Ask the physician which pulse changes are important and when to call about abnormal readings.

When taking pulse focus on the *rate* and *rhythm*. Simply, pulse rate is the *number* of beats per minute. Pulse rhythm is the *regularity* with which the beats recur. Ideal pulse is regular with one beat after another, evenly spaced. Abnormal pulse is uneven with too few or too many beats. As with temperature, normal readings vary from patient to patient.

Generally, normal pulse falls within the range of 60 to 100 beats per minute. This depends on the patient's age, physical condition, medication, and treatment.

You must learn pulse taking under the supervision of a physician or nurse. In this way you will be able to recognize your patient's special pulse characteristics.

A few words on pulse points. The point most often used in home care is at the wrist. Called the *radial* pulse, this spot appears on the wrist's outer edge, palm side up. Other points include the *brachial* (use for blood pressure readings—it's inside the bend of the elbow), the *carotid* (located on either side of the Adam's apple, a strong beat), the *femoral* (found on the inner aspect of the groin, and often used to measure pulse rate after vascular or coronary by-pass surgery). The physician or nurse will tell you which pulse point is best for your patient.

How to Take Pulse (See Figure 7).

1. Get a watch with a second hand.
2. Select a pulse point.
3. Use your three middle fingers and press firmly on the point. Important: Avoid the common mistake of pressing too hard, thereby blotting out the pulse.

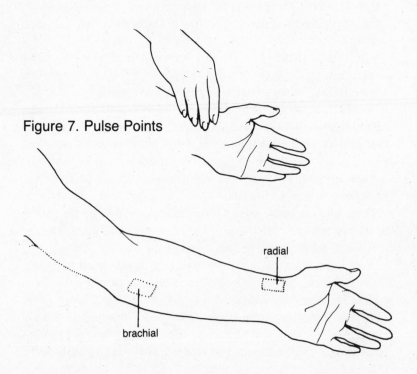

Figure 7. Pulse Points

radial

brachial

4. With your fingers on the pulse point and an eye on the watch count the beats felt for sixty seconds (or fifteen seconds and multiply by four). Note the rate and the rhythm.

5. Be sure there are no distractions and that the patient is quiet.

6. Record pulse rate and rhythm on Home-Health Chart.

Coronary By-pass Patients: Their Special Pulse Needs

In cases of irregular heartbeat the apical pulse should be checked. This pulse point is found under the left breast. Ask the physician or nurse for specific instructions.

Common Pulse Irregularities

• extra or premature beats: You detect a beat in addition to the normal rhythm; you feel one that comes earlier than expected.

• skipped beats: You do not feel an expected beat.

• thready pulse: You have difficulty getting a finger on the pulse. Beats may feel weak at all pulse points.

• atrial fibrillation: The physician will warn you that this can occur if your patient is susceptible. The pulse is very erratic and may be fast due to an overload of electrical impulses going through the heart. Consult with physician before or at the start of home care. This is not necessarily a medical emergency, but if it's a new development you should call the physician immediately.

How to Enter Pulse on the Home-Health Chart

Under the heading "pulse" include date, time of day, quality of pulse (strong and steady, thready, skipped beats, extra beats, etc.), rate per minute.

Vital Sign #3: Respiration

Respiration is simply the inhaling and exhaling of breath. For most people it occurs without thought or discomfort. For others it may be affected by underlying disease, pain, emotional distress, medication side effects, age, or room temperature extremes.

How to Take the Respiratory Rate

You will count the number of breaths your patient takes per minute. The average is between twelve to twenty times. Young children breathe about forty to forty-five times per minute. Both are normal ranges.

1. Get a watch with a second hand. Watch your patient's chest rise and fall. Each rise and fall counts as *one* breath. Or you can place your hand on the patient's chest or abdomen to feel the breaths.

2. Using the watch's second hand, count the respirations that occur during one minute. Record this number on the Home-Health Chart.

3. Observe the *quality* of your patient's breathing while checking the respiration rate. Indicate on the chart appropriate descriptions, such as easy, labored, painful, shallow, deep, breathing sounds, fast, slow.

How to Record Respiration on Home-Health Chart

Indicate the following information under heading labeled "respiration": respiration per minute, quality.

Respiration Alert

Call physician immediately if:
• patient is struggling to breathe
• patient has difficulty breathing and a fever
• patient has difficulty breathing, looks pale, and skin feels cold and clammy.

Vital Sign #4: Blood Pressure

Every second of the day blood travels through the vessels of the heart. While forcing its way through, it exerts pressure on the vessel walls. This is blood pressure.

Your patient's blood pressure depends on many things, such as age, health, strength of the heartbeat, and the elasticity of the vessels. Taking blood pressure is a skill that's best taught under the supervision of a medical professional. In this way you will learn your patient's average normal pressure. Then you will be able to detect abnormal rises and drops.

What about special equipment? You'll need a *stethoscope* and

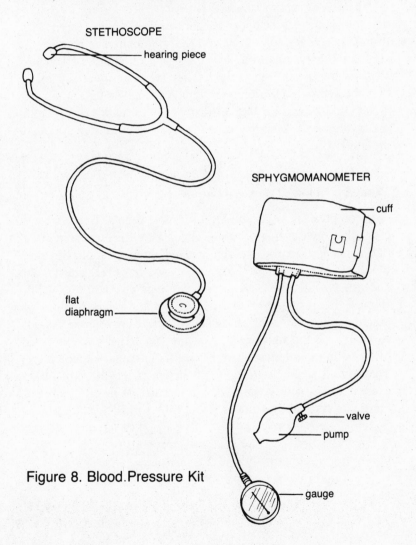

Figure 8. Blood.Pressure Kit

a *sphygmomanometer*. Most physicians recommend a stethoscope with a flat diaphragm for home-care readings. A dependable one costs $15 and up. Purchase at surgical supply store. There are several types of sphymomanometers. The least expensive and most convenient for home use is the *aneroid*. It has a round gauge with a meter attached to the blood pressure cuff. Ask the physician what he or she recommends for your patient. You may be advised to buy a *mercury* column or an *electronic* one. The mercury is similar to the type used in physicians' offices. It has a graduated scale usually positioned upright. They are often more expensive than the aneroid. Electronic sphygmomanometers do not require a stethoscope because they display readings automatically with digits or meters. Accuracy varies—the most expensive are often the most accurate.

What Do Blood Pressure Readings Mean?

Blood pressure is a stable sign for most people. Everyone has his or her own average reading which may fluctuate somewhat during the day. Stress, exertion, and certain medications can alter blood pressure readings. Most variations, however, are normal and usually fall within an acceptable range of 90/50 to 140/90. If these figures seem strange, don't panic. A few minutes of practice with a nurse or physician will clear up your confusion. Actually, the top figure is *systolic* pressure. That's the pressure of blood in the arteries when the heart's left ventricle contracts. The bottom figure is *diastolic*. It indicates the force of blood exerted against artery walls when the heart's at rest. The normal range for systolic pressure is 90 to 140, normal for diastolic is 50 to 90.

Finally, blood pressure that rises abnormally high is called *hypertension*, abnormally low, *hypotension*.

How to Take Blood Pressure

Use the following guide to supplement, not substitute for professional advice.

1. Ready stethoscope and sphygmomanometer. Be sure all air has been squeezed from blood pressure cuff. Remaining air can cause inaccurate readings. Reduce pressure in the cuff by turning the valve counterclockwise allowing air to slowly leak out.

2. Try to find the brachial pulse (see Figure 7) by palpation.

3. Place cuff securely around your patient's arm above the elbow crease. Adjust the cuff to fit. It should cover two-thirds of the upper arm. (Cuffs come in five sizes: infant, child, adult, larger adult, and thigh. The wrong size can lead to inaccurate readings.) The cuff should be tight enough so that only a finger can be slipped underneath.

4. Turn valve clockwise till it's closed. Squeeze bulb until reading rises above patient's average systolic pressure (usually 170).

5. Insert stethoscope into ears and place diaphragm on brachial point (pulse point inside elbow bend) before releasing air from cuff.

6. Once stethoscope is in place, keep an eye on the gauge (or mercury column) and gently open the valve just a bit to allow the gauge needle to move slowly (or the mercury to drop).

7. Listen through the stethoscope while watching the needle or mercury. Listen for pulse sounds. Record the first sound you hear; that's the systolic.

8. As the needle (or mercury) continues to drop, pulse sounds will continue. However, at a certain point they will disappear or muffle. Record the number when the sound disappears or muffles. That's the diastolic pressure.

9. Now open the valve completely to let pressure drop to zero. Remove cuff from patient.

How to Record Blood Pressure on the Home-Health Chart
Indicate time, systolic rate, diastolic rate.

How to Avoid the Most Common Blood Pressure Error
Beware of Ausculatory Gap, if you want accurate blood pressure readings. It happens when the gauge or mercury is not pumped high enough before the first (systolic) reading is taken.

The way to prevent this problem is to know your patient's average systolic—and always pump higher. For example, if your patient's average systolic rate is 170, the gauge must always be pumped above 170. Otherwise, readings can be underestimated. To guarantee accuracy, try several test readings before taking your patient's pressure.

Blood Pressure Alert
Call the physician in case of:

• a dramatic drop or rise in your patient's pressure compared to previous readings.

• a dramatic rise or drop in pressure after instituting medication or treatments

• a dramatic difference in blood pressure readings as the patient is lying down or sitting up.

5

How to Gain Health-Clue Savvy —and Be a Super Care Giver

This chapter is designed to help spare you some of the most apprehensive moments I experienced during home care—the moments when I wondered if a particular symptom was serious or not and debated whether to call the doctor.

On these next pages you will read about the most common physical and emotional signs home-care patients exhibit. Each health clue is identified and explained. You will discover which clues are cause for concern and which aren't. You will be told when to call the physician and under what circumstances to rush your patient to the hospital emergency room.

Get the most from these pages by reading them through at least once, then referring back to the specific clues as needed. One last thing: To make care-giving easier I have organized this section according to our senses of sight, smell, touch, and sound. Determine which sense you used to spot a certain clue; then check out the appropriate category. The clue should be explained and directions given. Good luck!

Health Clues to Detect by Observation

Activity

General
Watch for changes in your patient's normal activity pattern. They may occur suddenly or gradually. Consult physician about changes in any activities that you mark yes on the list below. Prompt action improves chances of reversibility.

YES	NO		YES	NO	
___	___	mental alertness	___	___	sleep pattern
___	___	memory	___	___	sex interest
___	___	use of language	___	___	responses to you
___	___	task performance	___	___	movement
___	___	vision	___	___	attitude
___	___	mood	___	___	hearing

Home-care emergency: Be alert to sudden activity changes that occur after administration of a new medication.

Body Movements

Your patient has his or her own style of movements such as a particular manner of walking (gait), facial movements, movements of extremities (arms, legs, hands, feet). Watch for any uncharacteristic actions.

Manner of walking (gait)
Watch for limping, unsteadiness, propulsive walk (patient leans forward while walking), balance problems, paralysis, arms and legs move out of sync.

Home-care emergency: Get professional help if you observe uncharacteristic actions. Possible causes: medication side effects, stroke, underlying illness, malnutrition.

Facial movements

Watch your patient's face to note expression and movement of facial features. Abnormal changes are excessive blinking, abnormal blinking movements (one eye blinks, the other does not), no blinking, fixed stare, loss of normal furrowing of forehead (forehead folds on one side only or not at all), drooping of eyelids and/or mouth, twitching, puffing up of cheeks, chewing noises, sucking.

Home-care emergency: Any unexpected facial movements demand immediate medical attention. Possible causes: medication side effects, stroke, nerve disorder, underlying illness, mental disorders.

Movements of extremities

Observe patient's arms, legs, and hands for abnormal movements. Changes to spot are:

• Tremors: These involuntary movements of a portion of the body are most common in the hands but can be seen in the arms and legs.

• Shaking: Usually seen as shivering or chills, shaking is most often associated with high fever or infection.

• Spasticity: A strong degree of muscle tone which interferes with the body's ability to stretch a muscle, spasticity can lead to shortening of muscles, ultimately causing contraction of an arm or leg. Possible causes are side effects to some medications, stroke and prolonged immobility.

• Restlessness: Frequent moving of an extremity or the inability of the patient to "sit still" may be emotionally induced by anxiety or other emotional disorders or the side effects of medications.

Home-care emergency: Seek professional assistance at sudden onset of any abnormal body movements.

Body positions

Nonverbal information about emotional and physical conditions is conveyed by the body's position. For example, a person curled up in bed may be in pain, anxious, or cold. A person sprawled across the bed may be overheated due to fever or room stuffiness. A person who stoops while sitting or standing may be in pain or depressed, and so on.

Home-care alert: To make sure that your patient is comfortable ask yourself: "Does he/she look comfortable?" If not, ask your patient why and correct the situation. Watch for natural movements. Joints should move easily. And keep your patient in a position that does not cause pressure sores. (See Chapter 3.)

Breathing Changes

Watch for changes in your patient's normal breathing pattern such as the rate of breathing (normal is between 12 to 20 breaths per minute) and quality of breathing (usually noiseless and easy; varies from patient to patient).

Hyperventilating

This is unusually rapid, shallow breathing, often associated with dizziness, lightheadedness, faintness, panic, and tightness in chest. Hyperventilating frequently shows in patients with a prior history of it. Or the bout may be preceded by emotional stress and anxiety. Continued hyperventilating is cause for concern. Call for medical help.

Shortness of breath

This looks like hyperventilation (rapid, shallow breathing), so how do you tell the difference? Hyperventilation frequently responds to reassurance or support; shortness of breath does not. Possible causes: respiratory disorders, lung disease, obesity (20% overweight), infection, emotional disturbances. Tip: To aid physician take your patient's vital signs before calling. (See Chapter 4.)

Home-care emergency: Breathing difficulties. Contact physician at once.

Snoring

Unattractive sounds coming from the patient's nose and mouth while sleeping are most often a sign of deep sleep, nasal blockage, or adenoids.

Home-care alert: Patients whose snoring interrupts their sleep may be hypoventilating. Consult physician.

Coughing

This is often beneficial to the patient because it rids the respiratory tract of overabundant and harmful secretions. For some it's a nervous habit; for others it can signal the start of a serious condition.

Home-care alert: Coughing is dangerous to the patient when it is persistent and exhausting and also dangerous to some post-surgery patients. Call for professional help if your patient does not respond to home treatment.

Home-care emergency: Call physician at once if cough is not easily stopped, produces bloody sputum or yellow or green sputum accompanied by fever, or is accompanied by pain and fever.

Wheezing

A sighing or whistling noise that happens during breathing, wheezing is often heard after a cold or respiratory tract infection. Home-care patients with allergies may wheeze; it is common in children, asthmatics, and patients with chronic pulmonary disease.

Home-care emergency: Call for professional help immediately if you observe combinations of these symptoms: wheezing, breathlessness, breathing difficulties, chest tightness, cough, or fever.

Sleep apnea

There may be periods of no breathing while patient is asleep. They can last from fifteen to thirty seconds and may be normal for some patients, abnormal for others. Sleep apnea is often seen in individuals with upper respiratory blockage and obese people.

Home-care emergency: Sudden onset of sleep apnea is reason for concern. In addition, it can cause sleep disorders and be potentially life-threatening for patients with heart problems.

Cheyne-Stokes respiration

Periods of rapid breathing followed by periods of slower breathing; this type of respiration is the most common form of periodic breathing. Cheyne-Stokes may be normal for some patients. However, it is of great concern if it is of sudden onset. Possible causes are cerebral disorders, thyroid disease, head injury, and medication side effects (especially morphine and barbiturates).

Home-care emergency: Cheyne-Stokes accompanied by high fever or headache is a medical emergency and can be a serious sign of central nervous system disease or a metabolic problem. Call for medical help at once, or get patient to hospital emergency room.

Kussmaul respiration

This type of respiration is characterized by periods of deep, regular, sighing breaths. The rate varies from slow to normal or fast, depending on patient.

Home-care emergency: Slow, deep breathing may indicate acidosis in diabetics. Medical emergency: Contact physician.

Painful breathing

Normal breathing is a painless process for most patients. Unless the physician indicates that a patient's condition is accompanied by painful breathing, know that breathing *with* pain is not normal. Seek medical evaluation.

Home-care emergency: Painful breathing with fever is a medical emergency. Call physician.

Home-care tip: The best way to describe breathing problems to the physician is to specify the rate of breathing (breaths per minute) and the pattern of respiration (short, fast, deep, shallow). Indicate if breathing problems are associated with pain or fever. Note if pain is increased by taking a deep breath.

Discharges

Discharge is the flowing out of liquidlike substances from the body's surfaces or openings. They fall into three groups: *purulent* (thick and creamy), *serous* (water), and *bloody*. In addition, discharges can be a combination of these types: bloody and watery, creamy and bloody, etc.

Home-care alert: Pinpoint the location of the discharge. Identify its type. Note the amount. Report to the physician.

Home-care emergency: These discharges are serious reasons for concern and demand immediate medical attention: discharge soaking through a bandage, bloody discharge, discharge with a foul smell, and accompanied by fever.

Bleeding

Look for abnormal blood loss rather than normal. (Normal: menstruation, minor cuts, gum bleeds after vigorous tooth brushing, etc.) Abnormal bleeding is an obvious process where blood oozes or spurts from a wound or body opening. Or bleeding may be hidden inside the body (internal bleeding) resulting from a wound, underlying disorder, or recent surgery.

Home-care alert: Know if your patient is susceptible to internal bleeding. If so, ask the physician what to expect and how to handle bleeding if it occurs. Patients at risk are people with blood disorders that impair clotting, chemotherapy patients, patients with ulcers, patients taking anticoagulants (blood thinners).

Home-care emergency: Any abnormal, significant flow of blood requires prompt professional attention. Call physician or get patient to the hospital emergency room.

Chills

Your loved one may appear cold and shiver. Possible causes are drafts, poor heating, inadequate bedclothes or bedding, fever from a wide variety of diseases and infections, aspirin given to bring down fever.

Home-care alert: Try to determine the cause of chills. Fever-induced chills are best handled by bringing down fever as quickly as possible. Contact medical professional for advice.

Home-care emergency: Shivering is the body's natural reaction to chilling cold. Shivering, when it occurs with fever, can cause the body temperature to rise—and this can be dangerous. Keep patient warm and try to bring down fever according to physician's instructions. If you cannot stop patient from shivering, call physician.

Dryness of Mouth

The most common cause is mouth breathing. Other causes are side effects of medication used for emotional disorders, gastrointestinal problems, muscle spasms, heart problems, hypertension, respiratory illness, and dehydration. Radiation therapy to the area around the salivary glands and chemotherapy can cause dry mouth, too.

Home-care alert: Mouth dryness is rarely a serious symptom in and of itself. To ease the problem, serve patient moist foods such as ice cream, juicy fruits, gelatin. Provide lots of liquids. Blenderized meals may be more comfortable to swallow. Avoid use of commercial mouthwashes because they contain two drying agents: salt and alcohol. Avoid cigarettes. If condition becomes severe, the physician can prescribe artificial saliva and other treatments.

Home-care emergency: Dry mouth is serious when combined with other symptoms. Get medical help immediately, or take your patient to the hospital emergency room if dry mouth occurs together with:

• breathing difficulties, nausea, vomiting, blurred vision, dilated pupils.

• pale, cold, moist skin; bluish lips, fingernails, and fingertips; dilated pupils; shortness of breath—may mean shock.

Ears

Observe any abnormal appearance or discharge from ear(s).

Home-care alert: Call physician as soon as you can if you spot these signs alone or in combination: tenderness behind ears, bleeding, discharge, and pain accompanied by fever.

Home-care emergency: Bleeding from the ear should be discussed with the physician immediately. Possible causes are ear infection, head injury, and perforation of the ear drum.

Eyes

Look for changes in the appearance of your patient's eyes.

Home-care alert: Report any of the following eye changes to the physician as soon as possible:
- change in color of the white
- prominence or bulging of eye
- drooping of one lid or both
- discharge from eye
- broken blood vessels or blood spot on white of eye
- eyes do not look ahead at the same time
- discoloration around the eye
- pain, burning, discomfort around the eye
- cloudy cornea
- eye excessively bloodshot for more than twenty-four hours
- sunken eyes
- abnormal eye movements
- vision problems.

Home-care emergency: Any sudden eye changes should be reported to physician. Sudden vision problems or eye pain are medical emergencies.

Fever

Be alert to sudden onset of fever (100°F. and above), persistent or high fever (103°F. and above in young children, 104°F. and above in adults). Fever often indicates the presence of infection, various blood disorders, malignancy, and other health problems.

Help the physician by noting other symptoms that accompany the fever.

Home-care alert: Call physician about any fever lasting more than twenty-four hours. Other signs to watch for: vomiting, coughing, painful breathing, infection, nausea, rash, headache, sore throat, breathing difficulties, abdominal pain, joint pain, confused thinking, chills, sweating.

Home-care emergency: Sudden onset of high fever demands immediate professional evaluation. In young children (under two) high fever can cause convulsions. Get medical advice about reducing fever.

Below normal temperature readings
Normal varies from person to person. (See Chapter 4).

Home-care alert: Below normal temperature, especially in patient who has not had below normal before, is reason for concern.

Home-care emergency: Rare. If you have any questions, it's best to call a medical professional.

Insomnia

You will recognize changes in your patient's normal sleeping pattern. Possible problems: difficulty sleeping, difficulty staying asleep, inability to get to sleep, restless sleep, or early waking. Insomnia is disturbed sleeping, not just the inability to sleep.

Causes? Anxiety (most common), depression, excitement, bladder problems, itching, overheated sickroom, overdressing, caffeine foods (colas, tea, coffee, cocoa, chocolate), heavy smoking, watching stimulating television before bed, reading stimulating material before bed, medication side effects. Infants and children may have sleeping problems due to teething or digestion difficulties.

Home-care alert: Discuss any persistent change in patient's sleep pattern with physician.

Home-care emergency: Sleep difficulties can be fatiguing and emotionally draining for the home-care patient. Problems lasting more than two days need professional assessment.

Intestinal Functions

Constipation

Note significant changes in your patient's bowel habits such as less frequent or difficult bowel movements that require straining because of hard stools or other problems. Some common causes of constipation during home care: bedrest, inadequate fluid intake, some medications.

Home-care alert: Report to the physician any constipation problem lasting three days or more.

Home-care emergency: Constipation *and* abdominal pain together are a serious combination that may indicate intestinal blockage. Call physician immediately.

Diarrhea

Note significant changes in your patient's bowel habits such as frequent, poorly formed, watery stools. Isolated bouts are often caused by intestinal problems, medication side effects, or radiation therapy.

Home-care alert: Frequent bowel movements persisting more than forty-eight hours are serious. Seek medical advice.

Home-care emergency: Call physician if your patient has diarrhea, associated with vomiting, bloody discharge, or fever.

Belching and flatulence

You may observe that excessive body gases are released orally and rectally by your patient. Possible causes are air-swallowing from too much sighing, some medications, eating quickly, drinking during meals instead of after, carbonated beverages, smoking, delayed bowel movements. Infants often swallow air while eating and during prolonged crying.

Home-care alert: Severe cases of belching or flatulence should receive medical attention.

Home-care emergency: Very rare.

Jaundice

Jaundice is a yellowing of the whites of your patient's eyes and skin. This abnormality shows when bile produced by the liver accumulates in the bloodstream causing certain parts of the body to turn yellow. Jaundice can also turn stools clay color or grayish white.

Home-care alert: This serious symptom may indicate liver, gall bladder, or pancreas problems or blood disorders. Discuss sudden appearance of jaundice with physician as soon as you can.

Home-care emergency: Sudden onset of jaundice accompanied by other symptoms such as vomiting, fever, and abdominal pain is a medical emergency. Get professional help fast.

Mental State

For the purposes of this section mental state is divided into two parts: *emotional changes* (changes in mood and behavior) and *mental changes* (changes in patient's alertness, ability to think clearly).

Emotional changes

Look for shifts in your patient's behavior and emotions. For example, uncharacteristic depression, euphoria, hostility, withdrawal. Such changes can be due to the stresses of illness, medication side effects, multiple sclerosis, hypoglycemia, and other underlying conditions.

Mental changes

Do you notice alterations in the way your patient thinks? Be alert to these problems: hallucinations, memory loss, disorientation, confusion, excessive drowsiness, difficulty concentrating, semiconsciousness, comatose signs.

Home-care alert: Many mental changes that occur during home care can be blamed on medication side effects. Call physician at once if mental changes occur after the administration of medication.

Home-care emergency: Mental changes are always a cause for concern. Seek professional guidance if you notice any of the following:

• mood change of sudden and intense onset
• mentally ill patients showing signs of recurring illness
• any patient who has become unmanageable and exhibits violent or excessively hostile behavior
• any patient not easily aroused from sleep or impossible to arouse from sleep
• any excessively drowsy or stuporous behavior.

Nose

Note abnormalities in the appearance and discharge from the nose.

Home-care alert: Watch for nosebleeds, mucous discharge, nasal stuffiness, snoring, and a clear, watery discharge.

Home-care emergency: Nosebleeds are rarely serious. However, they may be a grim sign if they occur after a head injury, in patients on anticoagulants, or if they interfere with breathing. If patient experiences a profuse and uncontrollable nosebleed, call physician at once.

Skin Changes

Skin can provide wonderful health clues. It takes an aware care giver to spot differences in the skin's normal appearance such as changes in color, texture, and odor. Make your observations while dressing, undressing, bathing, and touching your patient.

Moles

Change in the size or color of a mole or a sore that does not heal requires prompt medical assessment.

Flushing

A reddening of the skin that develops when blood travels to the face or other body parts such as usually is associated with good health or sunburn can have serious implications during home care.

Home-care alert: Areas of localized redness may be caused by drug side effects, nutritional deficiencies, underlying diseases, burns, vitamin (niacin) overdose, etc. They can also be due to emotional discomfort (blushing), indigestion, pregnancy, menopause (hot flashes), diabetes, epilepsy, chronic lung diseases, carbon monoxide poisoning, fever, or infection.

Itching

Irritation of the skin is rarely serious, but it can be annoying and in severe cases interfere with sleep. Itching is most often caused by dry skin. Other possibilities are hives, skin allergies, serum sickness, athlete's foot, lupus erythematosus, liver and kidney disorders, anaphylactic shock.

Home-care alert: The most popular cause of general itching, especially in the elderly, is dry skin. This is often due to excessive bathing. Ease discomfort of itching by applying body lotions and moisturizers after bath.

Home-care emergency: Itching is rarely an emergency. However, when it occurs in allergic reactions, it may be associated with respiratory difficulties, signs of shock, hives, or swelling. Call physician immediately.

Pallor

Paleness of the skin and mucous membranes (especially the lower eyelid), lips, and fingernails is often due to anemia (lack of sufficient red blood cells). Other causes are exposure to cold, which causes blood vessels at the skin's surface to constrict, heart or circulatory problems, perforated peptic ulcer, rheumatic heart disease, motion sickness, shock, and acute blood loss.

Home-care alert: Pallor alone is rarely a serious sign. But in combination with certain other signs (below), pallor can be very serious.

Home-care emergency: Extreme pallor in the following situations is a medical emergency and *demands immediate medical attention or an emergency room visit.*

• patient with history of peptic ulcer. Warning signs are ashen pallor with sudden onset of stomach pain, shortness of breath, pain in the shoulder, temperature, and pulse rise.

• shock: This is indicated by bluish lips and fingertips, shortness of breath, fast, weak pulse, cold clammy skin, anxiety, and unconsciousness.

• coronary thrombosis: The warning signs are severe anxiety, crushing pain in chest, cold sweat.

Rashes

Any inflammation or eruption on the skin can be a rash. Before calling physician about rash be sure that you know the answers to the following questions. In this way you can provide the medical professional with an accurate description.

1. Where is it located?
2. Does it itch?
3. Is the rash generalized over the body or localized at one spot?
4. Is the rash flat or does it have elevation?
5. Does the rash have lots of small red spots or is it one red area?
6. Does the rash look like a bull's-eye?
7. Is the rash blistering?
8. Is there associated fever?

Mouth and Throat Changes

Following are some tips to help you detect mouth/throat abnormalities.

• Look at mucous membranes (lining of the throat and mouth). They should be moist and smooth. Dryness may mean dehydration, excessive mouth breathing, or side effects of certain medication. If you suspect dehydration, call for professional advice as this can cause serious health problems.

• Look at tongue. It should be moist, smooth, and deep pink. Furrow or dryness may mean dehydration or excessive mouth breathing. Again, call physician if you suspect dehydration. Redness or swelling may be due to medication side effects or nutritional deficiencies. Brown or black tongue can occur after long antibiotic therapy. White patches may appear.

• Look at the back of the throat: The significance of the degree of redness can only be determined by a trained physician. Note the tonsils. Are they enlarged? Do they have any white patches? Are there any abscesses or other abnormalities in the throat?

• Look at the lips: They should be moist, smooth, and pink. Note very pale lips or bluish color. Dryness of the lips may be caused by chapping, excessive mouth breathing. Persistent cracking at the corners of the mouth may imply vitamin deficiency. Watch for unusual sores or growths on the lips.

Home-care alert: Mouth and throat observations are rarely medical emergencies. However, it's wise to discuss any abnormalities with the physician as soon as possible.

Home-care emergency: Rare. Any sudden appearance of growth, ulceration, or lesion that does not disappear within several days is cause for concern and requires prompt medical evaluation.

Stool Color

Stool, the material evacuated from the bowels, can reveal important health clues about your patient's condition. Normal stools are well formed, solid, medium brown masses. Watch for abnormal color.

Home-care alert: Abnormal colors include clay, green, mucous covered, black/tarry color, bloody, chalk, white discoloration or speckling, orange-red, yellow. Among the many causes are underlying health problems and certain drugs.

Home-care emergency: Certain stool colors indicate very serious health troubles. Get prompt medical assessment in the following instances.

• blood in stool: This is very significant and can signal internal bleeding or hemorrhoids.

• black/tarry stools: This is an abnormal condition suggesting internal bleeding or may occur as a side effect with patients taking iron supplements. Tip: You can use "hemoccult" slides to detect blood in stool. Buy at surgical supply store.

• clay-colored: This is important when associated with other signs such as jaundice, abdominal pain, dark urine; can imply liver, gall bladder, or pancreas disorders.

Sweating

You should be concerned with the frequency of sweating and the amount. It's often linked with menopause (hot flashes), fever, overheated sick room, overdressed patient.

Excessive sweating without apparent cause should be discussed with the physician as it may indicate an underlying disorder.

Home-care alert: Be sure your patient is not overdressed or that the sick room is overheated. Persistent sweating, especially in someone who is not prone to it, should be brought to the physician's attention.

Home-care emergency: Rare. By itself, sweating is not serious. However, persistent sweating could lead to dehydration. Give fluids. Call physician.

Swelling

Swelling means any enlargement on the body's surface or body part.

Home-care alert: Some people are susceptible to certain kinds of swelling, such as patients who are on birth control pills, pregnant, have vitamin B deficiency, premenstrual tension.

Swelling of specific body parts may be due to kidney problems (face, ankles), cirrhosis of the liver (abdomen, feet, legs), sickle cell anemia (hands, feet, especially in an infant). Get a medical evaluation of any sudden appearance of swelling.

Home-care emergency: One type of swelling that is life-threatening is swelling during anaphylactic shock. This is brought on by an allergic reaction to a foreign substance or food. Symptoms: giant hives, rapid pulse, breathing difficulties. This is a medical emergency. (See Chapter 10.) Call physician or get patient to the hospital emergency room immediately.

Pressure Sores

These are skin ulcers (also called bedsores and decubitus ulcers) that can appear after prolonged bedrest or wheelchair confinement. They can develop at the body's pressure points—elbows, shoulder blades, heels, buttocks, and other bony prominences that touch the mattress, bedding, or wheelchair.

If allowed to form and go untreated, pressure sores can turn into ulcerations that are very difficult to heal. They can become infected, even gangrenous. (For more detailed information about recognition and prevention, see Home Care Basic #5, p. 39.)

Urine Color

Consider this another clue in your care-giver's detective kit. Know that for most people normal urine color is straw.

Home-care alert: Watch for these abnormal colors. Note their significance. Call physician if you have any questions.

color	possible causes
very pale	Patient has been drinking lots of liquids; may have diabetes.
cloudy	May be caused by infection; natural chemicals present in urine.
milky white	Urinary infection.
blue or green	Usually not serious; often side effect of certain medications (Amitriptyline, Indomethacin)
red	Often a serious sign that indicates blood is present. Blood may be seen in patients who have kidney stones or are on anticoagulants. Call physician at once. Also, may be drug side effect. Some anticancer drugs (Adriamycin, Daunomycin) may be the culprits.
bright yellow	Often side effect of medication.
orange or dark yellow	May mean jaundice; high fever; inadequate fluid intake; side effect of medication.
tea-colored	Pus or bile may be in urine; glomerulonephritis after a strep infection.

Home-care emergency: Call for medical advice at once if urine shows up as red, brown, pink, or black. May indicate bleeding.

Weight Loss

Naturally this is not an unusual event during home care. Lost appetites, deteriorating conditions, poor eating habits, emotional distresses, the body's inability to absorb and digest foods, and other underlying health problems are likely causes.

Home-care alert: Any unexplained weight loss must be discussed with the physician.

Home-care emergency: Weight loss must be noticed and dealt with early to prevent health complications to the recovering patient. Lack of proper nutrients, fatigue, etc., can make recovery slow, if not impossible. Contact physician if you suspect problems. (See Chapter 6.)

Health Clues You Detect by Smell

Foul smells or unusual odors coming from your patient may signal a significant health problem.

Detect odors during close contact with your loved one, especially during feeding, bathing, dressing, undressing, and taking vital signs. In some cases, certain odors can warn of impending health crises and other serious conditions.

Body Odor

Fresh sweat is odorless. Infrequent bathing, however, allows bacteria on the skin to mix with sweat, thus forming body odor.

Home-care alert: Apart from its inelegant scent, body odor is rarely a serious health problem. In most cases it can be corrected with improved hygiene, especially to the body's warm folds: underarms, groin, rectal area.

Home-care emergency: Home-care patients with chronic kidney disorders could develop a urine smell on their bodies. This is a very rare but serious sign, because it suggests that the skin is taking over the function of failing kidneys. If you detect a urine smell (don't confuse with incontinence), call physician immediately or get patient to hospital emergency room.

Breath Odor

Most unpleasant breath odors are due to poor mouth hygiene, pungent-smelling foods (garlic, onions), alcohol intake, and smoking. Few mouth odors are cause for concern.

Home-care alert: Breath odors can be meaningful in people who have diabetes, respiratory disorders, and kidney problems. Get professional guidance if any occur.

Home-care emergency: Note breath odors in the following cases. They warn of a medical emergency. Call the physician immediately or get the patient to the hospital.

• diabetes: fruity, sweet smelling (like a several-day-old fruit bowl) breath can warn of diabetic acidosis—a potentially life-threatening condition.

• patients with kidney disorders: Urine smell on the breath is a very grave sign that may indicate that kidneys are not functioning properly. It may be associated with other signs such as breathing difficulties, diarrhea, vomiting, convulsions.

Discharge Odor

Certainly any foul-smelling discharges should be reported to the physician at once. Common sites include eyes, ears, wounds, nose, rectum, vagina, penis, mouth.

Home-care emergency: A foul-smelling, puslike discharge oozing from a wound or through bandages is cause for alarm. It may mean serious infection. Call for medical help.

Sputum Odor

Sometimes referred to as phlegm or mucus, sputum is the material discharged from the body's air passages—mouth and throat. Patients often remove sputum by spitting or swallowing.

Home-care alert: Nasty-smelling sputum can signal an underlying lung infection. This is a serious sign. Report to physician.

Home-care emergency: Foul-smelling sputum of recent onset accompanied by fever, coughing, and shortness of breath suggests a serious lung problem and needs prompt medical attention.

Stool Odor

The range here is from nearly odorless to extremely unpleasant. Stool odor is an important health clue, particularly in patients with diseases of the pancreas and digestion.

Home-care alert: Foul-smelling stool should be reported to the physician.

Urine Odors

Urine varies from aromatic, which is normal, to repulsive. Check out the chart below to help you recognize odors and their importance:

odor	*possible causes*
fishy	May indicate bladder infection.
foul odor	May indicate bladder or kidney infection.
fruity	Often indicates diabetes. Warning sign of diabetic acidosis; metabolic disorders

Home-care emergency: Urine produced by diabetics should be monitored closely. The best approach is to use a dipstick (Diastix) to check for the presence of ketones. Most diabetics are instructed in this technique. A monitoring system helps the diabetic to ward off health crises.

Vomitus Odor

Normally vomitus has a sour smell.

Home-care emergency: Vomitus mixed with blood is a medical emergency. Call physician at once or get patient to hospital emergency room. In rare cases vomitus can smell like feces. This may be caused by an intestinal obstruction. This, too, is a medical emergency.

Health Clues to Detect by Touch

Valuable information can be conveyed through your sense of touch.

• Use your fingertips to spot body subtleties such as lumps, bumps, and eruptions.

• Use the back of your fingers or the back of your hand to feel fever's presence.

• Use the palm of your hand to feel vibrations of heart activity and joints.

• Use your hands to gently reassure and comfort the patient.

Lumps

What do you do if you feel a small mass at some point on your patient's body? Call the physician and describe it as accurately as you can based on these guidelines: Is it hard or soft? Is it jelly-like? Is it irregular? How big is it? Is it freely moveable? Is it attached to underlying tissue? Is it tender to the patient when grasped?

Home-care emergency: Any lump or mass demands prompt medical evaluation.

Moisture

Wetness of the skin is rarely serious. However, in certain patients it can warn of impending health crises.

Home-care alert: Moisture or clamminess can be a symptom of shock, which is the body's inability to circulate blood to all its parts. This is life-threatening. Shock can result from drug side effects, diabetic acidosis, internal bleeding, kidney disorders, heart attack, or deteriorating health.

Home-care emergency: Shock is a medical emergency. Call physician immediately or get patient to the hospital if these signs occur: cold clammy skin, extreme pallor, drop in blood pressure, rise in pulse, shortness of breath. (See Chapter 10.)

Muscular Rigidness

Your patient may experience rigidness in his or her extremities and/or abdomen. You may feel a spasming or hardening in the muscles of your patient's limbs, stiff movement or loss of an easy style of movement. Or, you may feel a stiffness or hardening when you touch your patient's abdomen.

Home-care alert: For extremities: Onset of joint stiffness or lack of easy motion may be due to a variety of things. These include Parkinson's disease, stroke and side effects of antipsychotic drugs. Consult medical advisor.

For abdominal rigidity: When you touch the abdomen is there an unusual degree of hardness or stiffness? This is a cause for concern and should receive professional evaluation.

Home-care emergency: Rigidity in the extremities that occurs while patient is taking anti-psychotic drugs such as Haldol or Thorazine should be discussed with the physician immediately.

The combination of abdominal rigidity *and* abdominal pain is a very serious sign that needs immediate medical care.

Pulse Beats

Abnormal pulse can be a serious sign that requires immediate professional assessment. (See Chapter 4 under vital signs.)

Tenderness

You may notice that areas of your patient's body are tender to the touch. Often this is caused by a bruise or muscle soreness from exercise. There are times when tenderness is an invaluable sign, especially when linked with other symptoms.

Home-care alert: To describe tenderness accurately to the physician answer these questions: Where is tenderness located? How much of the body is tender? Are there other symptoms with the tenderness? Fever? Is there warmth or redness at the tender spot? Does the tender area pulsate?

Home-care emergency: Tenderness with other symptoms, especially fever, can be serious. Get prompt medical advice.

Texture

Watch for changes in the usual texture of your patient's skin. Dry skin is common during home care. Correct it by applying body lotion or moisturizer to the patient's skin after bath.

Home-care alert: Recognize crusting, coarseness, elevated rashes, small bumps, blisters, sores.

Home-care emergency: Rare.

Vibrations

Body vibrations usually mean cracking joints or pulse beats. (See Chapter 4 for complete information about pulse.)

Home-care alert: You may feel cracking or crunching vibration in your patient's joints. The knees are a popular site for this. Such vibrations may imply arthritis or bone damage.

Home-care emergency: Rare. Sudden appearance of decreased joint activity or cracking (with pain) needs professional attention.

Health Clues to Detect by Listening

The most efficient listening in health care is done through the physician's stethoscope. The sounds of the heart, blood vessels, lungs, and internal workings furnish excellent diagnostic clues.

Chances are that you've not been trained to use the stethoscope (except, perhaps, to take blood pressure). That means that you must rely on your ears to listen to your patient's body sounds and words. Be an alert listener. The tips to follow will show you how.

Body Sounds

You are listening for body sounds that are uncharacteristic of your patient.

Home-care alert: *New* and *persistent* body noises should be reported to the physician, especially in the following cases.

• respiration sounds: These are snoring, wheezing, high-pitched sounds when patient breathes in, and coughing and breathing difficulties.

• body sounds: These include belching, flatulence, and abdominal noises.

Patient's Speech

Listen for changes in your patient's ability to speak.

Home-care alert: Listen for slurred words, difficulty putting syllables together, nasal speech, stuttering. A new speech impairment such as difficulty finding words or incorrect use of words may be caused by drug side effects, stroke, high fever. Nasal speech is usually due to colds, adenoid problems, allergies, or flu.

Home-care emergency: The sudden onset of speech difficulties (except for nasal speech) is very serious. Call for medical guidance immediately as chances for reversibility of impairment improve with early detection and treatment.

Patient's Words

Recognize word choices and a style of speaking that are unlike your patient.

Home-care alert: The stress and anxiety of home care can make the best patient express frustration and seem irritable. Nonetheless, changes in your patient's use of language may signal mental changes. Possible reasons: medication side effects, high fever, stroke, mental disorders, brain cancer, head injury, brain tumor.

Call physician immediately if you hear any of the following:
- patient talks to him/herself
- patient uses language as never before (sudden use of profanity, hostile expressions, etc.)
- patient speaks, but makes little or no sense
- patient becomes threatening or menacing
- patient responds inappropriately to your questions

Home-care emergency: Sudden or gradual appearance of changes in the way your patient expresses him/herself are very serious. This is a medical emergency. Call physician immediately.

Responding to Your Patient's Complaints

Up until now we have been concerned with what you, the care giver, observe through your senses. Now let's focus on the patient's own complaints and what to do about them.

Abnormal Bleeding

Complaint: Patient complains of bleeding.

Action: Pinpoint the site of bleeding. Determine if the bleeding is expected; if unexpected, assess the amount of blood and seek medical evaluation. If bleeding results from an injury, try to stop it (see Chapter 10).

Call physician immediately about unusual and/or profuse bleeding or take patient to hospital emergency room.

Loss of Bladder Control

Complaint: Patient complains of urinating involuntarily.

Action: May be complication of illnesses such as neurological disease, diabetes, aging process, side effects from medication, or certain infections. Call for medical advice as soon as possible if this symptom occurs suddenly and unexpectedly.

Complaint: Patient says that there's pain, burning upon frequent urination.

Action: This is a very uncomfortable combination of symptoms. Before calling physician determine whether or not your patient has fever. Fever associated with frequent urination, burning, and pain can indicate kidney problems or other infection. Then call for medical evaluation.

Loss of Bowel Control

Complaint: Patient complains of involuntary bowel movement.

Action: This is rarely an emergency. Possible causes are neurologic disorders, gastrointestinal illness, diabetes mellitus. Requires complete medical assessment to find cause.

If loss of bowel control is linked with numerous bowel movements the consequences can be serious—dehydration and metabolism problems. If condition lasts more than twenty-four hours, call physician.

Loss of Power

Complaint: Patient complains of lost coordination, movement difficulties, sudden weakness in limb (arm, leg).

Action: Loss of coordination is most often due to neurological disorders, circulatory problems, trauma, and side effects of certain medications. Get professional advice promptly as this is a very serious sign.

Loss of Sensation

Complaint: Patient says he or she has lost feeling in a specific body area.

Action: Possible reasons: brain disorders, spinal cord or nervous system disorders; can occur in diabetics or after injury. This sign requires immediate medical evaluation. Warning: Know that loss of sensation can reduce or eliminate a person's ability to feel pain and temperature extremes. Take precautions to avoid injury.

Swallowing Difficulties

Swallowing difficulties can interfere with nutrition if the underlying problem does not have a ready solution. Any swallowing difficulties lasting longer than twenty-four hours should be reported to the physician as soon as possible.

Complaint: Your patient may say that he or she has pain in the mouth, discomfort in the back of the throat, or pain in the chest when swallowing.

Swallowing difficulties are most likely to occur when patients have had them before, or in cases of surgery of the larynx, esophagus, or throat. Disorders such as multiple sclerosis, certain types of stroke, allergic reactions, and throat inflammation can cause swallowing difficulties.

Action: Determine the cause of the swallowing problem. Here are the most common.

• inflammation: By itself this is little cause for worry. If accompanied by fever that persists more than forty-eight hours, seek medical guidance.

Home-care alert: Trouble swallowing with coughing or respiratory difficulties increases the risk of aspiration. This is a serious condition where food or liquid may be breathed into the lungs causing pneumonia, suffocation, even death. Call physician at once if swallowing problems are joined by coughing spells and respiratory problems.

• blockage: Obviously, any food or foreign object stuck in the throat can interfere with swallowing. To dislodge perform Heimlich Maneuver (see Chapter 10) or get your patient to the nearest emergency room immediately.

• allergic reactions: Some people are allergic to certain foods or substances that can affect the ability to swallow. Contact with these substances can cause swelling in the throat and in severe cases be life-threatening.

Know your patient's allergies so that in most cases offending substances can be avoided. If you suspect allergic reaction, stop patient from using the troublesome item and get medical help.

Home-care emergency: Anaphylactic shock is a medical emergency. It can occur in patients who are hypersensitive to certain drugs, foods, and insect stings. The allergic response can be so overwhelming that in minutes convulsions, loss of consciousness, and death can occur. Prime offenders: insect stings (wasps, bees, hornets, yellow jackets) and penicillin. Most patients know of their susceptibility and take precautions accordingly. At other times you must act quickly to get medical help or take your patient to a hospital emergency room. Symptoms of anaphylactic shock: giant hives all over the body, tightness in the throat, breathing difficulties, rapid pulse, and rapid drop in blood pressure. An "ANA Kit" should be available for susceptible patients in anaphylactic shock emergencies. It can be purchased at a surgical supply and contains life-saving equipment. Consult physician.

Hearing Disturbances

Complaint: Your patient may say that he/she:
• hears ear noises
• has ear pain
• has hearing loss.
Action:
• ear noises: These "sounds" usually puzzle physicians. Many disappear as suddenly as they came. However, ringing noises can be a significant signal of drug overdose—especially aspirin, quinine containing drugs, some antibiotics, and a condition called Ménière's Syndrome. Get medical evaluation.
• ear pain: Pain in the ear can occur at the ear or be referred pain from another site such as the neck, throat, or jaw. Pain can be mild, moderate, or severe; there may be an uncomfortable sense of fullness in the ear. Seek physician's help if earache occurs by itself or is joined by fever, bleeding, discharge, hearing loss, balance problems.

• hearing loss: Any unexplained hearing loss demands immediate medical evaluation. A medical emergency exists when loss of hearing is associated with these symptoms: balance difficulties, loss of sensation on part of the face, swallowing difficulties.

6

How to Help Your Patient Eat for Recovery

Your patient is home ill. What can you do to be sure that the food he or she eats is packed with get-well nutrients? Read this chapter. Carefully. I'm not pushing fad diets—there's no place for them in home care. And I'm not talking about nutritional secrets—they simply don't exist. I am talking about common-sense eating. And foolproof ways to tempt the weakest appetites.

Your home is the best place for this because it's more conducive to eating than a hospital or institutional setting. After all, you can prepare your patient's favorite meals, serve food when he or she wants to eat, and stimulate appetite with tenderness and caring. What hospital can do that? Not one.

So what's your job in all of this? Simply to guarantee that your loved one gets enough vital nutrients and calories to maintain strength, prevent weight loss (or gain), and rebuild tissues affected by illness or treatment. How? Read on.

Your Eat-for-Recovery Guide

When a person's ill it means that he or she must take in more essential nutrients than when well. And that means more protein, carbohydrate, fat, vitamins, minerals, and water. How do you serve them? No one food supplies them all. So scientists have developed the Basic Four—four food groups, each with unique home-health benefits designed to supply good nutrition. What are they? Meat/fish/poultry/beans; vegetable/fruit; milk/cheese; bread/cereal.

Serve a variety of foods from each group to improve your patient's chances for optimum emotional and physical health. Also, check out the home-health benefits I have listed with each group. Knowing them will enable you to emphasize certain foods to meet your patient's special needs.

(Note: If the physician has prescribed certain diet restrictions for your patient, you will have to make some adjustments in the Basic Four. These will be discussed later in the chapter.)

Meat/Fish/Poultry/Beans

Food choices: beef, veal, lamb, pork, poultry, fish, shellfish, dry beans, dry peas, soy beans, lentils, eggs, seeds, nuts, peanut butter.

Daily servings: 2.

Home-health benefits: Vary choices, as each has special nutritional advantages. This group is an invaluable source of protein. Protein repairs tissues affected by illness and treatment, and maintains strength, enabling patients to better withstand surgery, chemotherapy, radiation therapy, immunotherapy, and infections.

Vegetable/Fruit

Food choices. The best *vitamin C sources* are grapefruit, oranges, citrus fruit juices, cantaloupe, raw strawberries, broccoli, green pepper, brussels sprouts, sweet red pepper. The best *vitamin A sources* are dark green and yellow vegetables such as broccoli, carrots, collards, kale, spinach, winter squash; some fruits, especially apricots, cantaloupe, mango, pumpkin.

Daily servings: 4.

Home-health benefits: Vitamin C is essential for healing wounds and strengthening the walls of blood vessels. It's crucial to the bedridden or wheelchair-bound patient because it also helps prevent skin breakdown that can lead to pressure sores. Vitamin A, known as the "anti-infective" vitamin, helps the body resist bacterial and viral infections and helps keep inner body linings healthy. There is scientific evidence that vitamin A helps in the body's protection against cancer, particularly in tobacco users.

Milk/Cheese

Food choices: milk and most milk products—whole, skim, low-fat, evaporated, and nonfat dry milk, buttermilk, yogurt, ice cream, ice milk, cheese, cottage cheese, process cheese foods and process cheese spreads.

Daily servings: adults, 2; children under nine, 2–3; children nine to twelve years and pregnant women, 3; teens and nursing mothers, 4.

Home-health benefits: These are calcium-rich foods that aid in proper functioning of the heart, muscles, and nerves; they help coagulate blood during bleeding and maintain hardness of bones and teeth.

Bread/Cereal

Food choices: whole grain and enriched breads (check labels), including cooked and ready-to-eat cereals, pasta, rice, rolled oats, baked goods with enriched flour or corn meal, crackers.

Daily servings: 4.

Home-health benefits: Important sources of B vitamins, iron and protein. Prime protein source for vegetarians. A variety of foods from this group can help with proper functioning of nerves, encourage normal appetite, good digestion, prevent anemia, and promote energy.

Common-Sense Eating Tips
Serve more of these foods:
- whole grains
- fruits and vegetables

- low-fat dairy products
- poultry, fish, legumes, nuts
- vegetable oil and polyunsaturated spreads.

Serve less of these foods:
- egg yolks
- high-fat dairy products
- fats such as butter, shortening
- alcohol
- sugar and high-sugar foods.

A Few Words on Fad Diets and Vitamin Supplements

- Again and again dieticians and nutritionists from major hospitals told me: The best nutritional gift you can give the convalescent home-care patient is a well-balanced diet.
- Clearly, fad diets are out of the question. They fail to supply the essential nutrients most patients need.
- It's worth noting that vitamins are not innocuous substances. Doses of vitamins greater than ten times the Recommended Daily Allowance are considered toxic. For example, large amounts of vitamins A and D taken over long periods can accumulate in the liver and interfere with its proper functioning. Too much vitamin C can create a vitamin C dependency. The result: If excessive vitamin C is suddenly stopped signs of vitamin C deficiency may appear.

Important point: If you are thinking of giving large doses of vitamins to your patient, check with the physician first.

- Vitamin Tip: Are you worried that your patient is not getting enough vitamins and minerals in his or her diet? Try this safe solution. Provide a once-a-day multivitamin. These supplements contain 100% of adult daily requirements. (For children, there are special multivitamins.) Their use can prevent vitamin overdose—a common risk when people gobble down the latest cureall vitamins touted in the media.

Serve Breakfast to Fight Illness

It is a healthy idea for your patient to have a morning meal during his or her convalescence in order to help maintain strength and weight. When the morning meal is missed repeatedly important calories, proteins, vitamins and minerals needed for healing may be missed too—and not recouped at other meals.

Encourage your patient to eat breakfast. I know this isn't always easy. Saggy appetites and finicky tastes don't help. My advice: Don't treat breakfast like breakfast. Instead, offer your patient tempting taste sensations that depart from the mundane. The list below is a smattering of the possibilities. As one dietician told me: "Anything goes for breakfast, as long as it's nutritious."

Treats to Get Your Patient to Eat
a Nutritious Breakfast

• fortified milkshakes (see recipes at end of chapter)
• Carnation Instant Breakfast (commercial breakfast supplement from your supermarket)
• plain, low-fat yogurt or cottage cheese topped with fresh fruit and/or chopped nuts, raisins, granola
• English muffin or pita bread pizzas (top muffin or pita with tomato sauce and favorite cheese, heat in oven)
• peanut butter on crackers or whole wheat with fresh fruit
• favorite soup
• grilled cheese or melted cheese on toast.

My Secret Weapons to Lift Sagging Appetites

Illness can perform a disappearing act on appetite. Beyond that some medications, radiation therapy, and chemotherapy can change taste and smell.

I can't emphasize enough the importance of fighting—and winning—the battle of lost appetites. Your patient must not be allowed to lose weight (unless a weight-loss diet is prescribed) or nutrients. Muster your energy and imagination to help your loved one eat for recovery!

If you're faced with a less-than-willing eater, try these hints.

• Consider consistency when preparing meals. Some people are turned off by mushy foods, others by crunchy ones. Avoid consistencies that may repel your patient.

• Alcoholic beverages stimulate appetite in some people. Check with physician to see if some brandy or wine before meals is all right.

• Sweetness perks some palates. If appropriate, try sweet fresh fruits, raisins, dates, jams and/or syrups as toppings. On the other hand, some people develop an aversion to sweets while they are ill and/or after certain treatments. In such cases, try to reduce the sweetness of things. For example, add more milk to milkshakes and reduce sugar added to recipes.

• Serve small portions. They're less intimidating.

• Serve appealing food. Don't present food in a messy, jumbled way. Use garnishes such as watercress, orange slices, carrot sticks. For children (and adults who are young at heart!), make fun-food shapes. Use cookie-cutters to make animals, star shapes. Take thin strips of meat, cheese, fresh fruits, or vegetables and write the letters of your child's name. Each letter eaten can score a point toward winning the "eat-for-recovery" game.

• Serve small meals more often, as if they were doses of medication. Provide one "dose" every hour or two. This can be as simple as offering a fortified milkshake (see end of chapter for recipes), a cheese slice, fresh fruit—anything nutritious.

• Liquids are often easier to down than solids. Serve milk and juices.

• Leave snacks near patient for munching—just in case an urge strikes.

You Can Add Calories and Protein to Meals
—and Not Increase Portion Size

Do you want to build your patient's strength? Does your loved one have little desire to eat? Is he or she losing weight? What can you do to solve these problems—without piling lots of intimidating eats on the plate?

• You can add protein by mixing diced or ground meat into vegetable dishes, sauces, casseroles, soups; serving peanut butter on crackers, fresh fruit, or celery sticks; adding skim milk powder (good protein source) to hot or cold cereals, scrambled eggs, meatloaf, baked desserts; mixing canned fish (tuna, shrimp) or hard-boiled eggs into sauces or serve over rice, noodles, toast.

• You can add calories by mixing mayonnaise (100 calories per tablespoon!) into salads, spreading on sandwiches; breading meats such as fish, chicken; providing high-calorie but nutritious snacks such as dried fruits, ice cream, milk shakes, cheese, and crackers; adding whipped cream (60 calories per tablespoon) to fruit, hot chocolate, baked goods, Jell-O.

So Your Patient's a Vegetarian...
What About Extra Protein and Nutrients?

Your best bet is to serve a variety of cereal grains. One protein complements the other, increasing the value of both. Some ideas: Offer sunflower seeds (good sources of protein and vitamins) as a snack; mix brewer's yeast (good source of B vitamins) into soups and cereals.

Try these helpful books for vegetarians: *Eating for the Eighties* (a complete guide to vegetarian nutrition), by Janie C. and Neil J. Hartbarger, Philadelphia: The Saunders Press, 1981; *Laurel's Kitchen* by Laurel Robertson, Carol Flinders, and Bronwen Godfrey. Berkeley, California: Nilgiri Press, 1976.

How to Help Your Patient Eat
Despite Nausea and/or Vomiting

The good news is that this is possible! Of course, you'll want to pinpoint the reason for your patient's distress. Some possibilities are medication side effects and aftereffects of radiation therapy or chemotherapy. (Unexplained nausea and vomiting lasting twenty-four hours is cause for concern. Call physician at once.)

The physician may recommend a special diet during this difficult time. In addition, he or she may prescribe an antiemetic (antinausea drug). This medication is usually taken one-half hour before meals and can restore a dulled appetite. Also (with doctor's permission) try these ideas:

• Small, frequent feedings.

• Clear, cool drinks are often easy to sip.

• Your patient can suck on small cubes or ice chips if drinking is difficult. Make ice cubes from nutritious fruit juices such as lemonade. Tip: Avoid liquids at meals. Ask patient to drink them thirty to sixty minutes before eating.

• Provide carbonated beverages such as ginger ale.

• Encourage your patient *not* to lie flat immediately after eating. If he or she is tired, it's better to sit. If your patient must lie down, elevate head at least four inches higher than feet.

• Know that for some patients pickles or lemons may ease nausea.

• If there are specific times when your patient feels nauseated don't plan favorite foods at these times. He or she may develop negative associations to them and ultimately avoid them.

Does Your Patient Have Mouth, Throat,
or Chewing Problems?

With a bit of planning you can help your loved one enjoy nutritious, tasty meals despite oral difficulties.

Milk, for example, is a superb protein source. Serve it flavored with chocolate or other syrups. Use it liberally in soups, puddings, gravies, and custards. Cook cereals in milk rather than water. Make a fortified milk beverage (see recipes at the end of this chapter).

Meat can be made chewable. Cook meat or poultry slowly to make it more tender. (High temperatures make it tough.) Sprinkle minced meat over soft vegetables, noodles, pasta, or rice. Prepare stews using chicken, fish, meat and/or vegetables. Your butcher can grind meat—lamb, veal, pork—to be made into a loaf. Cook slowly and well.

Eggs—as in egg salad, scrambled eggs, or omelettes—are a tasty, easy-to-chew alternative.

Fish can be broiled, baked, or poached. Cold fish salads of tuna or salmon are inexpensive and easy to prepare.

Fruit that is soft and succulent is best sliced. Biting into a fruit such as a peach may be difficult for some patients.

Cheese, a palatable protein-rich choice, can be eaten as is or shredded over macaroni or rice. Cottage cheese can be mixed with crushed fruit or vegetables, or it can be sprinkled over noodles.

The list goes as far as your imagination and common sense allow.

What about patients who have mouth soreness or dryness? This is a common side effect of certain drugs, radiation therapy, and chemotherapy. To make eating more comfortable remember to:

- avoid serving acid or very salty foods
- avoid hot spices such as chili powder, pepper
- use straws rather than a spoon or serve in cup
- serve fortified milkshakes (see recipes)
- eliminate cigarettes and alcoholic beverages
- serve cold, soothing foods such as frozen ice cream, yogurt, Jell-O, add ice to drinks.

Taste Perception . . . Sometimes It Changes
. . . What to Do?

Some treatments can make an individual's taste sense go haywire. Numbness in the mouth or bitter or metallic taste sensations may develop. Some foods just won't taste right. Naturally, you must check with the physician to be sure this is a drug or treatment side effect and not the sign of a more significant problem. When taste problems are caused by treatments such as radiation or chemotherapy there are ways to make your patient's life more pleasant.

• Reduce strange tastes by increasing intake of liquids (water, ginger ale, etc.) or serving foods that leave their own tastes such as hard candies and sweet fruits.

• Add wine, beer, or mayonnaise to sauces to enhance their taste. Note: Alcohol *evaporates* when cooked. This advantage should be considered if your loved one is on an alcohol-restricted diet.

• Add poultry or fish to cream soups for additional flavor, protein.

• Food tastes better to some patients when served cold or at room temperature: experiment.

Turn Your Blender into a Good Nutrition Machine

Lots of nourishing foods can be prepared in liquid form. For some patients they may be a delightful change of pace. For others, with chewing problems and oral difficulties, they may be a necessity. Either way, use any type of broth, milk, juice, or water as a base. Try adding fresh vegetables, fruit, ice cream, yogurt, protein powder, eggs, wheat germ to create a variety of concoctions.

Stews can be blended into a delicious soup. Of course, blending certain foods takes a little know-how. You can make things blend more smoothly by:

- warming ahead of time when blending potatoes, vegetables, or meat
- slicing meat into fine pieces before blending.

An excellent source of inspiration is the *Blender Cookbook*, Better Homes and Gardens, Des Moines, Iowa: Meredith Corp., 1971.

The Best Way to Get Your Patient to Follow a Restricted Diet

If your patient is on a restricted diet, the secret to making it appealing is to understand the diet thoroughly and adapt it to your patient's tastes and life-style. More often than not physicians handle restricted diets by giving their patients a list of foods to eat or delete—and hope for the best. Under these circumstances many patients leave the doctor's office and try to follow the prescribed diet, although they are frequently unable to do so effectively.

To solve this problem consult a *registered dietician*. This professional has been highly trained to help you and your patient understand the purpose of the diet and adapt it to personal tastes and life-style. Dieticians can offer suggestions for food preparation and advice to finicky eaters as well as provide resources for you to get additional nutrition information.

To find a dietician, ask the physician or nurse for a referral or call your local hospital, social service department, public health department or visiting nurse service.

Be sure that the person you select is a registered dietician (R.D.). This title indicates that the individual has passed a nationwide test which qualifies him or her to provide nutrition and diet counseling.

Hints to Make Your Patient's Restricted Diet Work!

In addition to getting information about your patient's diet from the physician or dietician, you may want to go one step further. There is an excellent book that explains restricted diets clearly and intelligently, and it contains basic recipes that are adapted to many different types of diets. Check out *Just What the Doctor Ordered*, by Harriet Wilinsky Goodman and Barbara Morse, New York: Holt, Rinehart and Winston, 1982. Two other books to consider: *The New Nuts Among the Berries*, by Ronald M. Deutsch, Palo Alto, California: Bull Publishing Co., 1977, and *Jane Brody's Nutrition Book,* by Jane E. Brody. New York: W.W. Norton and Co., 1981. Both are excellent general nutrition guides.

In the meantime, I have included the most common restricted diets below with explanations and tips for their use.

Soft-Solid Diet
This diet is often prescribed when a person has difficulty chewing or digesting. Two fine books to help you plan soft-solid meals are *The Soft Foods Cookbook*, by Anne S. Chamberlin, Garden City, New York: Doubleday and Co., 1973, and *Hamburger Cookbook*, by Betty Crocker, New York, Golden Press, 1977.

Mechanically Soft Diet
Here, food must be of a liquidlike consistency. It's ideal for patients who lack dentures, have mouth inflammation, or have had oral surgery or have wired jaws. You will be expected to provide frequent feedings of blenderized foods or liquids. In addition, you may be able to provide nutritious prepackaged formulas. Check with physician. See end of this chapter for more information.

Ulcer Diet
This diet may be recommended when a person has a peptic ulcer, duodenal ulcer, or other disease of the upper gastrointes-

tinal tract, such as gastritis. Your patient will probably be asked
to experiment with small amounts of a variety of foods to see if
they cause gastric upset. Avoid caffeine (coffee, tea, colas), alcohol, black pepper, chili pepper.

It's usually best to serve your ulcer patient three balanced meals
a day. And he or she should sit up at least one hour after meals
to avoid gastric acid reflux.

In the past, high-fiber (roughage) foods have been excluded
from this diet, but there is no evidence that these foods really
cause irritation. Lettuce, nuts, and fruit skins may be eaten, but
should be chewed carefully and mixed well with saliva.

Liquid Diet

Does your patient have difficulty keeping food down? This
diet will probably be suggested because fluids are often more
easily tolerated than solid doses of food. Offer liquids a little at
a time. (This diet may be ordered before certain diagnostic tests.)
Here's a choice of beverages from each of the three possible
liquid diets.

clear	full	bland
water	clear liquid	full liquid diet
ice	*and* milk,	except tea,
tea	soups, plain	coffee, colas,
coffee	yogurt	meat soups,
carbonated drinks		broths,
clear broth		seasoned soups
apple, cranberry juice		
Jell-O (any kind except with fruit)		

Low-fat/Low-cholesterol Diet

Actually, fats are an essential part of our diet. So why restrict them? Because too many Americans get too much of this nutrient, which makes for excess calories and increases the risk of heart disease.

The purpose of this diet is to improve the *quality* of fat your patient eats. For example, it's better to eat fewer saturated and more unsaturated fats. That is, eat less visible fat (as seen in meat and butter, butterfat products, and whole-milk dairy products) and eat more polyunsaturated vegetable oils. Use oils such as safflower, corn, soy, or cottonseed. (Among other bonuses these oils provide the body with essential fatty acids.)

The low-fat diet tries to lower elevated levels of cholesterol and other lipids in the blood in an effort to reduce heart disease. This is the type of eating style the physician will recommend: Limit beef, lamb, pork, to three three-ounce portions per week. Use only skim milk and lean meats, fish, poultry (without the skin), and veal. No shrimp, butter, whole milk. Limit total fat intake to two tablespoons a day. For detailed information about low-fat diets write to your local heart association or to the American Heart Association, National Center, 7320 Greenville Ave., Dallas, Tex. 75231.

Fat-restricted Diet

Your patient may need this diet so that certain body organs, such as the pancreas, gall bladder, and liver, are allowed to rest. You will receive a complete list of forbidden foods. Restriction ranges from mild to severe. Some samples are no whole milk, cream, cheese, cake, gravy, sauces, oil, mayonnaise, butter.

Chemotherapy and Radiation Therapy Diets

It is essential that patients undergoing chemotherapy or radiation therapy eat well-balanced meals. In this way they can maintain strength to better handle treatments and help the body build new tissues and cells. Be sure your patient gets a variety of foods from the Basic Four food groups detailed earlier in this chapter. Emphasize protein-rich foods. Add high-calorie foods when necessary, particularly if your patient is losing weight.

It's worth noting that for most cancer patients secondary diet restrictions are dropped until treatments are finished. Why? Because many physicians believe that it is more important to fill a cancer patient with nourishing food to maintain weight and energy than to worry about diet restrictions for a secondary health problem. For an excellent source of recipes and tips for better nutrition during cancer treatment, read *Eating Hints*, issued by the National Cancer Institute (see end of this chapter for address).

Diabetic Diet

A person who has diabetes has elevated blood-sugar levels and an undersecretion of the hormone insulin. This triggers a chain reaction in the body, leaving it unable to metabolize carbohydrates, fats, and proteins. Furthermore, the underproduction of insulin, if unchecked with special diet and/or medication, can cause serious complications such as diabetic ketoacidosis, coma, and death. Over the long term diabetes can lead to premature coronary heart disease, kidney failure, poor circulation, blindness, and stroke.

With this in mind, you'll want to be sure that your diabetic patient's diet is planned carefully. Unfortunately, few physicians are able to do this. That's why I recommend that you and your patient see a dietician to discuss the diet and its restrictions as they apply to your patient's individual likes and dislikes. This diet counselor should be in touch with the physician so that he or she understands your patient's unique health needs. It is a very bad idea to depend solely on a preprinted handout given out by medical professionals. The physician or dietician will supply a complete list of foods to avoid and to eat.

In addition to the meal plans you will receive, here are some important tips for diabetic individuals to remember.

• Maintain ideal body weight. Weight loss is necessary to bring down sugar levels.

• Avoid skipping meals.

• Understand the word "dietetic." It is used to mean many things, including low fat, low salt, low calorie and low sugar. Diabetics are most concerned with sugar and fat content.

• A product that claims it is sugar-free may not be. Read labels carefully for chemical sugar substitutes: sorbitol, xylitol, and manitol. They contain carbohydrates and when taken in excess raise blood-sugar levels.

• Sugar should not be one of the first five ingredients listed on a food label. Watch out for sugar and sugar words, such as words ending in "ose" (dextr*ose*, malt*ose*, mann*ose*, etc.)

• Limit fruits and fruit juices to four servings a day. Fruit has natural sugars. Too much fruit can aggravate a diabetic's condition as much as eating a candy bar. Juices should be unsweetened, canned fruits always packed in water. Whole fruit is preferable to juice.

• Watch fat intake. The reason: Diabetics tend to develop coronary artery disease. As a preventive measure serve your patient a poly-unsaturated, low-saturated fat diet. That is, select polyunsaturated oils and lean meats instead of fatty meats. Choose polyunsaturated margarine instead of butter.

• Limit intake of egg yolks to three times a week. Watch out for eggs "hidden" in products such as egg noodles, canned soups, etc. Limit red meat, increase intake of fish, poultry (without the skin), and veal.

• What are Food Exchanges? This is a confusing term. Simply, foods are divided into six groups: milk, vegetables, fruit, bread, meat, and fat. Foods are categorized into groups according to portion size and their amounts of carbohydrate, protein, and fat. The diabetic is told to select foods within these groups so that he or she gets the total number of calories needed without actually counting calories. This enables the diabetic to eat the correct amount of carbohydrates at the same time each day without eating the same food. Careful carbohydrate intake is important when an individual needs to regulate insulin and/or diabetes.

High-fiber Diet

A high-fiber or high-roughage diet is often indicated for people with uncomplicated diverticulosis, irritable bowel syndrome, and certain types of constipation. You increase your patient's intake of whole grain breads and cereals, fresh vegetables, and fruits high in fiber. The daily addition of a bran supplement to the diet is a simple, inexpensive way to increase fiber intake.

Lactose-restricted Diet

Some people have trouble absorbing or digesting a milk sugar called lactose. (Note: Not everyone has the same reaction to the same quantity of lactose. It is an individual thing and reactions are unique to each person.)

Lactose is found predominantly in milk and dairy products. It may already exist in foods or be added to them. Read labels carefully to detect lactose.

Generally, an intolerance to lactose is inherited, but it can occur in combination with certain medical treatments—particularly abdominal radiation and some antibiotics.

Naturally, you will be given a list of foods to avoid serving your patient. Some of the most common are cheeses, except those aged ninety days, all milk products, cocoa, most chocolate drinks, cream, desserts filled with cream or custard, yogurt. Be careful when preparing foods containing dry-milk solids, gravies, dips or sauces made with milk or cream, any dressings, or food with dairy products added, powdered coffee, or cream.

Low-sodium Diet

A low-salt eating style is usually prescribed for patients who have hypertension, congestive heart failure, renal disease, or edema, or are on adrenocortical therapy. The physician will tell you how much salt to eliminate from your patient's diet. Restrictions range from low to severe. Regardless of how strict the diet is these foods should be avoided: salt in any kind of cooking or at the table, canned vegetables, meat, fish or soups unless prepared *without* salt, frozen peas, frozen lima beans or frozen prepared foods, fruits preserved with benzoate of soda, salted fats, bacon and bacon fat, cheeses except for salt-free cheeses. Beware of these sodium-containing compounds: monosodium glutamate, sodium chloride, disodium phosphate.

Even your drinking water can be a source of too much salt. If your local water supply has a high sodium content cut down on it or avoid use of locally bottled carbonated beverages, wines, etc. In severe restrictions drinking water may have to be distilled or supplied by bottled water from other areas. Also, know that water softeners add sodium.

You will find many helpful recipes in these two publications: *Cooking Without Your Salt Shaker*, published by the American Heart Association (contact your local chapter); and *Secrets of Salt-Free Cooking*, by Jeanne Jones, San Francisco: 101 Productions, 1979.

Radical Methods of Feeding Special Patients

Suppose your patient cannot receive food by mouth. In the past, he or she would have been hospitalized. Today it's possible to manage such patients at home. How?

Tube Feedings

Perhaps your patient has had head or neck surgery, jaw fracture, oral radiation therapy, or trauma to the oral area from a stroke, accident, or malabsorption problem. Clearly, each of these can prevent normal eating. However, complete nutrition can be given through a tube that is passed through the nose (nasogastric tube) or a tube passed directly into the stomach (gastrostomy tube). Into the tube is poured a liquid formula or blenderized diet that can meet a person's nutrition needs for a time.

True, this method can be handled at home, but it's important to know that there are possible side effects. Some patients may experience diarrhea, nausea, or vomiting. To spare your loved one as much distress as possible you must follow the special instructions from the physician or nurse. Also, tube feeding equipment should be handled in a highly sanitary way to diminish the chance of infection.

For more information about tube feeding write to the companies that supply the formulas used for it. Mead Johnson & Co. and Doyle Pharmaceutical are two. See the end of this chapter for addresses.

Parenteral Nutrition

This is an intravenous method of feeding a person. It can be used in the home for patients who suffer from chronic diarrhea, certain bowel diseases, malignancies, intestinal obstructions, malabsorption problems, or side effects from radiation or chemotherapy. Most often it is instituted in the hospital.

In most situations the physician will insert a large-caliber needle into a vein. A highly nutritious mixture is administered to the patient in this way. You will be given special instructions to care for the site where the needle enters the skin. One of the most troublesome and potentially dangerous side effects of this technique is infection at the needle-site. Therefore, it is very important to follow professional instructions for sanitary care.

Recipes

Here are some nutritious liquid delights that may come in handy when you cannot get a finicky eater to eat, or when your patient has little appetite or chewing and swallowing difficulties. These recipes are not intended to substitute for a well-balanced diet.

Rather they may supply extra calories, protein, and nutrients to patients not interested in or having difficulty eating conventional meals. (The following has been adapted from *Eating Hints— Recipes and Tips for Better Nutrition During Cancer Treatment.* Excerpts in this chapter appear with the courtesy of the National Cancer Institute. The booklet is an excellent source of nutrition advice for cancer patients or anyone who is home ill. Write for a free copy to the Office of Cancer Communications, National Cancer Institute, Bldg. 31, Rm. 10A18, Bethesda, Md. 20205.)

Fortified Milk

This recipe doubles the protein in each cup of milk.

1 quart milk, homogenized or 1% low-fat
1 cup instant nonfat dry milk

Pour liquid milk into deep bowl. Add dry milk and beat slowly with beater until dry milk is dissolved (usually less than five minutes). Refrigerate. The flavor improves after several hours. Makes one quart.

calories: 275 per cup with homogenized milk
195 per cup with low-fat milk

High-Protein Milkshake

1 cup fortified milk
1 generous scoop ice cream
½ tsp. vanilla
2 tbsp. of patient's favorite syrup (chocolate, butterscotch, etc.)

Pour all ingredients into blender. Blend at low speed about 10 seconds. (For low-fat diets be sure to use low-fat milk and ice milk.)
calories: 485 per recipe

Fruit Shake

½ cup favorite frozen fruit (strawberries, blueberries, etc.)
1 scoop ice cream
½ cup milk

Blend all ingredients until smooth. For low-fat diets use low-fat milk and ice milk. For sugar-free diets substitute unsweetened fruits. Diabetics must make appropriate adjustments.

calories: 355 (with frozen strawberries) per recipe

Nutritional Formulas and Preparations

There are good diet supplements on the market that are useful when your patient has difficulty chewing, swallowing, or eating solid foods. The physician or dietician can provide information about these products.

However, to get you started, consider the most accessible preparation: Carnation Instant Breakfast. You can find this powdered beverage in the supermarket. It's highly nutritious and can be served as an occasional substitute for meals or as a snack. Just add powder to the milk and you have a meal in a glass!

Furthermore, there are companies that manufacture special nutrient-packed liquid formulas. These can be "eaten" as is or used as an ingredient in shakes.

For more information you can write the companies that manufacture these products. Two of the best resources are Mead Johnson and Co., 2404 Pennsylvania St., Evansville, Ind. 47721 and Doyle Pharmaceutical Co., 5320 W. 23rd St., Minneapolis, Minn. 55416. Among the products put out by Mead Johnson are Sustacal and Isocal; by Doyle Pharmaceutical, Meritene and Citrotein. Recipes are also available from the manufacturers.

More Recipe Books

The Book of Soups, by Robert Ackart, New York, Dolphin Books: 1982 (contains over 200 soup recipes).

Cookbook for Boys and Girls, by Betty Crocker, New York: Golden Press, 1977 (useful when the kids must do some of the cooking).

The Milk-Free/Egg-Free Cookbook, by Isobel S. Sainsbury, M.D., New York: Arco Publishing, 1974.

One Pot Meals, by Margaret Gin, San Francisco: 101 Productions, 1979 (large selection of easy-to-chew, simple-to-prepare meals).

Recipes for Diabetics, by Billie Little, New York: Grosset & Dunlap, 1981.

7

Care-Confidence: Taking Care of Your Patient After Surgery

Let's take a few steps back for a moment to presurgery. Naturally, you'll want a highly qualified surgeon to perform the necessary procedure. To find one ask your family physician or consult knowledgeable friends. No matter how you go about this, be sure that when you do you check his or her credentials—thoroughly!

How? Refer to the special directories found in most libraries that list surgeons' backgrounds. Find the *Directory of Medical Specialists*, the *American Medical Association Directory* and the *Directory of the American College of Surgeons*. Look up your surgeon's name to see if he or she is board certified. This means a surgeon has passed special boards in a chosen specialty (for example, general surgery, neurology, obstetrics). The surgeon may be listed as "diplomate" of a particular board. Then, confirm that this doctor is listed as a "fellow." That is the proof that your surgeon possesses top ethical standards and professional abilities. It is indicated by the initials F.A.C.S. In addition, you should consider the quality of the hospital where the surgeon has privileges and the rapport between the patient and surgeon. Both should be top-notch.

After you select a highly qualified surgeon, it's time to face the next most important issue concerning surgery: realistic expectations. As one surgeon told me: "Patients must know the limitations of the surgery recommended for them. They must not expect miracles to be performed when they are not possible."

I believe that a good surgeon explains things simply and realistically. Your job is to listen carefully so that you understand the surgery's benefits and risks. One more thing: Whenever surgery is prescribed, seek a second opinion. Unnecessary surgeries are performed every day. Be convinced that the procedure recommended for your loved one is the right choice.

How to Handle Surgery's Most Common Aftereffects

As care giver you will want to be prepared for your patient's return home from the hospital. To be sure, he or she may encounter some discomforting aftereffects. These will seem less upsetting if you offer understanding and support. Be prepared for experiences of the following type.

• loss of hair: Many surgical procedures call for shaving the surgical site and often a large area around it. Your patient may be disturbed to see a once hairy area now baby smooth or stubbly. The good news is that hair grows back. The bad news is that this takes time—and meanwhile, itching and changed body image can be bothersome. Tip: Sprinkle baby powder on the affected area to ease itching. Reassure your loved one that this uncomfortable stage passes quickly.

• fatigue: Expect your patient to return home exhausted. Most do. This may be frightening to some—especially if they felt fit before the surgery. Rest assured that this fatigue is a normal part of convalescence. It's caused by a constellation of things: the wear and tear of anxiety before and after surgery, the poor eating and sleeping habits that are so often part of hospital life, and the physical trauma of the operation. Your patient will not feel like his or her old self for a while. This is an individual thing, so ask the surgeon how long it will take your patient to feel "whole" again.

• change in body image: Most surgery leaves behind a scar, and some surgeries are so radical that they remove body parts such as breasts or limbs. Your patient will have his or her own reaction to the scar: For some it's a cause for considerable grief.

My advice: Discuss the type of scarring to be expected *before* the surgery is done. Some scars are hairline thin and fade quickly. Some remain angry red souvenirs for a long time. You may want to ask the surgeon to consider the cosmetic needs of your patient—if it is possible to do so.

If your patient is very self-conscious about the incision or amputation, be sensitive to these feelings. Your reaction and acceptance may be crucial to his or her self-esteem. Never show disapproval or disgust, no matter how unsettling the site of the scar is to you. Not only would this be emotionally painful to someone you love, it could make self-acceptance twice as hard, if not impossible.

• strange sensations around the incision: Don't be surprised if your patient mentions disagreeable feelings around the incision site. The light touch of clothing may now feel "funny" or uncomfortable against the wound. Maybe there is numbness. Ask the surgeon about these new feelings. In most cases they are perfectly normal. Clearly, the cutting of nerves and skin during surgery can alter an area's natural responses. For most patients it takes six months to a year for normal sensation to return. There are cases when it never does.

Physical Activity After Surgery— How Much Is Too Much?

Once again, this can only be determined by the nature of your patient's surgery. Be sure to get explicit instructions from the surgeon about limitations if any are imposed. For example, the physician may say that during the first two weeks at home lifting heavy objects, driving a car, or having sex are out of the question.

On the other hand, your patient may be encouraged to resume some activity. It's your job to encourage as much movement as the physician allows. Mobility and activity can help prevent complications such as clotting and pneumonia—both health risks after extended bed-rest.

Pain Watch—What Should You Expect? What Should You Do?

Clearly, this depends on the type of surgery done. For many, pain is not a significant feature upon returning home. Chances are your patient's most intense discomfort was felt during the forty-eight hours after surgery. Painkillers of varying strengths may have been given.

I suggest that you ask the surgeon how much pain to expect during your patient's recuperation. In this way you can spot abnormal pain and seek medical guidance when necessary. *Important: Any pain accompanied by fever and/or nausea, vomiting, reddening, discharge, tenderness, or warmth at the wound site is cause for concern. Call physician at once.*

Another consideration is your patient's tolerance for discomfort. An annoying ache to one person might be considered a major misery to another. Try to get a realistic perspective on the kind of pain your patient feels. Let me add, too, that some people use pain as an excuse for dependency and incessant complaining. Perhaps it's hard for you to imagine that someone you love would do such a thing. Just remember that illness can bring out the child in all of us. And that child can be needy, fearful—and demanding. Be prepared.

There are nondrug ways to handle pain. True, there is pain that will only diminish with the help of painkillers; yet there are lighter discomforts that can be handled without medication. One way is to splint the uncomfortable area by propping pillows up against it during movements or coughing. Another is to know that pain is often aggravated by stress. Many things can make your patient tense—guilt, self-consciousness, worry about prognosis, and so on. Help your patient relax by recognizing the problem and discussing it. Still another source of relief for your patient is distraction. Sometimes a preoccupation with pain makes it seem worse. Turn on the television, radio, record player—anything to get your loved one's mind off the situation. Important: *Persistent discomfort should be discussed with the physician.*

Hints You Need to Care for the Surgical Wound

Does your patient have sutures (stitches) still in place? Ask the physician how to care for them. There are different types of sutures, each with special care considerations.

Generally, patients are told to shower regularly and to keep the wound area clean. You may be advised to dip a cotton swab in hydrogen peroxide, then rub the suture line gently to diminish crusting. If so, don't go digging—be gentle. Or you may be told to keep the site dry.

Dressings are another story. Some people return home without any—just a bare incision. Others have a gauze pad and adhesive tape covering the wound. Again, get explicit instructions about dressing changes. In the case of complicated ones, th physician may send a visiting nurse to your home to change the dressing and teach you and/or the patient how to do it.

Naturally, you must keep an eye on the wound. Healing may be uneventful—or you may see significant signs that must be reported to the physician immediately.

Call the physician about the incision if there is redness, increased pain, new oozing drainage, foul smell from wound, area becomes hot to touch, increased swelling, fever, nausea, vomiting, bulging at the wound site, bleeding. Don't wait for a combination of symptoms—any *one* is reason to worry.

Call the physician about the dressing if it is full of pus. This may indicate infection or bleeding under the surface. *Call physician at once.*

Once sutures have been removed, your patient may say that there's tightness or itching at the scar. This is definitely a natural reaction. To lessen discomfort, gently rub cocoa butter or lanolin cream over or around the scar. Ask physician or nurse for their suggestions, too.

Healing should be a prime consideration. Vitamin C is necessary to enable your patient to heal properly. You may want to emphasize vitamin C-rich foods in your patient's diet. (See Chapter 6.)

Finally, two caveats: First, coughing may cause undue stress on the wound site. Call physician if your patient's coughing persists. Second, the incision site is new skin. That means it never has seen sunlight. Tell your patient to be careful when exposing this area to the sun. Protect it by covering the scar tissue with a strong sunblock. If this is not done, a severe sunburn can occur, ultimately accentuating the incision's appearance.

Be Prepared for Twenty Post-Surgery Emergencies

Here are twenty surgeries and their possible home-care emergency consequences. There are a multitude of other procedures that could not be included here because of space limitations, but these are among the most common. If you have any questions about your patient's recent surgery, call the surgeon for advice.

Amputation

In the event of removal of a limb, call physician if:
- temperature rises or limb feels unduly hot
- any place inside dressing causes discomfort or pain for more than twenty-four hours
- the cast loosens so that patient can feel stump move around
- mechanical parts of a temporary limb break or become loose.

For your information: Phantom pain may occur after this surgery. This is pain in the missing part. It's a natural occurrence.

The physician can prescribe stump exercises to alleviate this condition. Ask a medical professional for guidance.

For more information write Medic Publishing Co., P.O. Box 89, Redmond, Wash. 98052. They publish two excellent pamphlets: *Amputee's Guide Above the Knee* and *Amputee's Guide Below the Knee*.

Appendectomy

When the appendix has been removed, call physician if there is:
- pain, swelling, or drainage at wound site
- fever
- vomiting, diarrhea

Arterial Surgery

This involves withdrawal of a clot or scraping inside an artery. Call physician if there is:
- fever
- swelling, redness, drainage at wound site
- blueness, cramping, or coldness in arm or legs
- loss of sensation.

By-Pass Surgery

This relatively new type of surgery is being performed with increasing frequency. Unfortunately, many patients return home with insufficient information about their conditions. That's why I'm including a detailed description here. (For additional information write for a helpful booklet called *Moving Right Along...After Open Heart Surgery*, c/o Pritchett & Hull Associates, Inc., Suite 110, 3440 Oakcliff Rd., N.E., Atlanta, Ga. 30340.)

What Did the Surgery Do?

The physician decided that your patient's coronary arteries (the arteries that supply the heart with nutrients to function) had deposits of cholesterol and other body fats. This condition, called atherosclerosis, causes the arteries to narrow and in some cases blockage results. The trouble is that this blockage can lead to heart attack or a painful angina condition.

During the operation the surgeon removes a portion of the saphenous vein from the leg. (Sometimes an arm vein is used instead.) One end of the vein is grafted to the heart's aorta; the other is attached to the coronary artery below the blockage. The result: Oxygen-rich blood can now travel from the aorta through the graft, by-passing the blockage and feeding the heart muscle necessary nutrients.

Are There Special Considerations for the Home-Care Patient?

Most definitely. Your loved one will return with two incisions, one on the chest and one on the leg. The long chest scar will eventually fade to a hairline. The leg scar will fade, but be more noticeable than the chest incision.

Follow the surgeon's instructions for incision care. Your patient may be told to take a medication such as Tylenol to ease discomfort. Also, there may be leg swelling as an aftereffect of the surgery. A heating pad set on "low" applied for twenty minutes four times a day may reduce it. Be sure to check with the physician first.

Your patient may experience many emotions. Fear is most common. He or she may fear additional complications, such as a heart attack. Your reassurance and support is needed at this time. Exhaustion is also to be expected. It is a natural result of any surgery, especially this one. Profound fatigue may alarm some people who did not feel ill before the procedure was done. Arrange for two twenty-minute rest periods daily for the first week or two during home care. This doesn't mean that your patient has to go to bed. It does mean he or she must relax.

Remind your patient that it's important to take one day at a time and not to get discouraged during the early recovery stages.

Perhaps your patient will be depressed. This, too, is natural. Lots of emotional energy is expended to handle anxieties about surgery and afterwards. Tearfulness and crying are not unusual. Tempers may be short. Some people even experience temporary memory loss or difficulty concentrating. These are normal reactions considering the extent of this type of surgery. Expect easy days and tough ones. You'll cope better if you remember that most of these symptoms disappear at the end of four to six weeks, the average recovery period. Ask the surgeon for an activity guide. Generally, during the first couple of weeks nothing more demanding than setting and clearing the table, short walks, or dusting furniture should be done. After four to six weeks, jogging, swimming, and fishing are usually possible. But check with the physician to be sure.

When to return to work should be decided at the end of four to six weeks. The choice made depends on the demands of the job and the patient's condition. Warning: *Premature return to work or unprescribed activity can lead to serious health complications.*

As care giver you can help your loved one diminish stress during recovery. For example, discourage visitors during the first two weeks at home. Rest is crucial to successful recovery. Be sure that your patient gets eight to ten hours of sleep per night. Staying up late should be put off for a while.

Sex, another source of concern for most by-pass patients, is discussed in greater detail in Chapter 9.

By-Pass Surgery Alert: Call physician if there is:

• redness at the incision site
• more pain than before
• foul smell or thick drainage
• fever
• increased swelling
• coughing, chest pain, and/or drastic change in vital signs.

Cataract Surgery

Here, the eye's lens is removed to eliminate spots that impair vision. Most often tiny sutures are used to close the incision. Sometimes dissolvable sutures are used. A bandage is worn over the eye for several days.

If your patient is a cataract patient, the best home-care medicine you can give is preventive. Your patient must avoid being poked in the eye as this can cause serious damage to the vulnerable surgery site. Be sure patient avoids crowded subways and buses, and all places where the presence of lots of people increase the potential for accidents. Because your patient has temporary vision impairment, his or her balance may be off. Falls are possible, so be alert. Make your house safe by being sure there are no open closets or doors that a person can walk into.

If your patient wears glasses, watch to see that he or she does not stick the stems into the eyes when putting them on. If drops have been prescribed, be sure that *you* administer them. An occasional patient has been known to bump the surgical wound with the dropper, causing serious eye injury. Never press on the eyeball. When applying drops, keep this tip in mind—press on the cheek bone below the affected eye to allow drops to flow inside the lower lid.

Above all, use common sense. Your patient should not lift heavy furniture or perform any activity that can result in an accident until the eye heals. On the other hand, there is no harm in using the eye for activities such as watching television and reading. It will not cause injury.

Surgery is not the end of cataract care. Since your patient's lens has been removed, proper focusing is impossible. Therefore, glasses or contact lenses should be prescribed by the doctor to return the eye to normal function. One ophthalmologist told me, "People shouldn't fear contacts after cataract surgery. Most are afraid they can't handle them. That's bunk. Many people do a lot better than they expected."

Cataract Surgery Alert: This procedure rarely causes complications during home care. Your patient may experience some discharge, scratchiness, or redness of the eye. These are all temporary disorders. Call physician, however, if there is increased discomfort or other alarming symptoms.

Colon Resection

In this operation the affected portion of the colon is cut and the remaining healthy portions above and below the removed area are stitched together. The removal of a tumor is the most common reason for this surgery. If the tumor is benign, your patient is likely to return to a normal life after recovery. If the tumor is malignant (cancerous) the surgery and post-surgery treatments may be more complicated. Radiation therapy, chemotherapy, and/or a colostomy and special diet may now be necessary.

If the tumor was benign, call physician in the event of:

• irregularities at the incision site such as redness, increased pain, new oozing drainage, foul smell from wound, localized heat, increased swelling, bulging at wound site, bleeding, fever, nausea, vomiting

• fever, nausea, vomiting, and/or diarrhea.

If the tumor was malignant ask physician for specific instructions.

Craniotomy

This procedure involves opening the skull to remove a brain tumor, treat an aneurysm—weakened wall of an artery—or to correct complications from an injury. The incision's location depends on the position of your patient's tumor, aneurysm, etc. In many cases recovery is rapid and the incision heals quickly.

However, malignant tumors can be very serious. They require radiation therapy and other treatments. Recovery depends on the ability of the surgeon to remove the cancer and the area affected.

When no malignancy is involved, home care means rest and a well-balanced diet. Fatigue is the most common aftereffect. The incision site heals relatively quickly, and in most cases there is little limitation on activity.

Call physician in case of:

• any irregularity at the incision site
• a return of any symptoms experienced *before* surgery
• changes in mental status or muscular movement.

Dilation and Curettage (D & C)

This procedure involves scraping the lining of the uterus for therapeutic, diagnostic, or abortive purposes. Call physician if there is:

• fever
• severe abdominal pain
• vaginal bleeding heavier than a normal menstrual flow.

Note: Sexual activity may be resumed in most cases after staining ends. Ask physician for advice.

Gall Bladder Surgery

One caveat here: The removal of the gall bladder often leaves behind an abdominal incision that may be uncomfortable during early recovery at home. Ask the physician for painkillers. Your patient will be told about the amount of mobility and activity allowed. Inspect the incision site daily for abnormalities.

It's possible that the physician may prescribe a low-fat diet for your patient at first. In most cases, though, gall bladder patients can return to foods they could not tolerate after the condition developed.

Call physician if there are:

• any irregularities at the incision site
• fever.

Gastrectomy

This surgery is often recommended for peptic ulcer patients. When part of the stomach is removed a special diet is often prescribed. Ask physician for guidance.

Call physician in the event of:
- any irregularities at the incision site
- vomiting or diarrhea.

Heart Valve Surgery

It is sometimes necessary to repair an individual's heart valve or replace it with an artificial valve or tissue valve. Either way the surgery is intended to help the heart to pump more efficiently. Your patient may feel improved after the surgery because his or her physical symptoms are alleviated. However, most patients must wait a few months before they experience the advantages of this procedure. One reason is that the heart needs time to recover from the additional work it has been doing. As a result the physician may prescribe certain medications and life-style adjustments.

In addition, anticoagulants (blood thinners) may have been prescribed for your patient. Because these drugs can cause problems for some people with certain types of valves, it's important that your patient keep appointments for regular blood tests. Watch out for these signs of bleeding: tarry stool, pink or red urine, severe headaches and abdominal pain, blood in vomitus that resembles coffee grounds. Do not administer aspirin or any medication containing aspirin including Bufferin, aspirin with codeine, Alka-Seltzer, Excedrin. If any dental work or surgery is planned, tell the doctor that your patient is taking anticoagulants.

Finally, after valve surgery your patient may be more susceptible to an infection of the heart lining called *bacterial endocarditis*. This can scar or destroy the heart valves. It can occur after dental work, some surgeries, and undetected infections elsewhere in the body. It can be averted if your patient is given antibiotics before procedures and, sometimes, afterwards. Consult your medical advisor for guidance. For incision information see By-Pass Surgery alert, p. 154.

Hemorrhoidectomy

In this operation veins in the anal and rectal area are removed. Call physician if there is:
- fever
- constipation
- difficulty urinating
- considerable bleeding from the operated area.

However, you should expect some slight bleeding from the anus for a few weeks. Ask the surgeon how much bleeding is normal so you may detect abnormalities.

Hernia, Hiatus

This type of surgery is called for when the opening, or hiatus, through which the esophagus passes enlarges sufficiently to push the stomach against the chest. Call physician in the event of:
- irregularities at the incision site
- feeling that food has stopped beneath the breastbone
- diarrhea persists (may occur for a brief time).

Hysterectomy

Too many of these operations are performed unnecessarily. Therefore be sure that the reasons for a hysterectomy are carefully considered—and that your patient has received at least two opinions.

Your patient will experience some physical and possibly emotional changes after this procedure. The kind of changes will depend on the extent of the surgery. For example, after a hysterectomy menstruation stops and pregnancy is impossible. If the ovaries are removed menopause will start immediately. This can mean hot flashes and other symptoms. There should be no changes in your patient's sex life or breasts.

Call physician in case of:

- irregularities at the incision site.
- hot flashes
- vaginal bleeding exceeding a slightly bloody discharge
- abdominal cramps or a change in bowel habits.

Mastectomy

I am appalled by the number of surgeons who treat the removal of a breast as they would the removal of a gall bladder or an appendix. It is an intensely emotional experience for many women and it should be handled with sensitivity and concern. Indeed, many women have difficulty articulating their true feelings after this surgery. Some may feel they now are "damaged goods." Others may experience a loss of femininity. Many worry about rejection from their husbands or lovers. This is compounded by the fact that the medical diagnosis is cancer. In short, mastectomy patients must face a change in body image as well as the consequences of their illness. It is imperative that women receive psychological support at this time. If this support, caring, and reassurance can come from you, the care giver, fine. But in most cases mastectomy patients benefit greatly from the help of other women who have had similar experiences. Your patient can rediscover her potential with the compassionate support of self-help group members. Contact your local American Cancer Society, hospital, YWCA, family services, or self-help hotline. Also try the National Self-Help Clearinghouse (see Chapter 2; also Chapter 9).

As for the physical side of home care, your patient's arm on the affected side is susceptible to infection and swelling because lymph nodes and lymph vessels have been removed. Call physician at once if you see any of these signs of infection: the arm become red, unusually hot; the arm becomes unusually hard or swollen. Watch out for any irregularities at the incision site. Note: Blood pressure should not be taken on the affected arm.

Ostomy

In this procedure, a tiny piece of the small intestine is brought out surgically through the abdomen to by-pass abnormalities in the colon (colostomy), ileum (ileostomy), and urinary tract (ileal conduit, also sometimes called urostomy). Although each procedure is unique, they do have one important home-care consideration in common, the *stoma*. This is the new exit for body waste (fecal matter or urine) and appears on the abdomen to replace the no longer available colon, rectum, or ureter. After surgery a drainage appliance is fitted to the outside of your patient's body to catch existing waste material.

There are a few important things you must be aware of. First, it is crucial that the stoma site be *selected before* surgery. Why? To be sure that it is in a comfortable location, and that, in the case of obese patients, skin folds do not obstruct the stoma.

I have seen new ostomy patients struggling to manage their stoma- and appliance-care at home. The most common reasons for the struggle are poor hospital instruction and the fact that visiting nurses are not always knowledgeable in the proper care for ostomy patients.

Help your loved one to avoid this hassle by finding an *enterostomal therapist*. This is a registered nurse who has had special training to help ostomy patients adjust physically and psychologically to their new body image and functions. Some hospitals provide this nurse automatically. Many do not. To locate the nearest therapist contact International Association for Enterostomal Therapy, 505 N. Tustin Ave., Suite 282, Santa Ana, Calif. 92705.

Beyond that, your patient may need the additional emotional support of self-help groups to adjust to his or her new body image.

Indeed, sex lives can be altered by certain ostomies. Colostomy in men, for example, can cause impotence. Of course not all ostomies have such a profound effect on their patients. (For more information on sexual functioning see Chapter 9; for more information about self-help groups write to United Ostomy Association, 2001 West Beverly Blvd., Los Angeles, Calif. 90057.)

As for home care, call the physician if there are any irregularities at the incision site. In most cases there is at least one incision and one stoma site. After surgery the stoma is larger than it will be a year later. While it's in the process of shrinking, be sure to check frequently that the appliance fits. Get professional help in case of:
- skin redness and irritation on and around stoma
- appliance's not fitting properly
- ileostomy's failure to function properly for about three hours and/or cramps.

Stoma care tips: Every ostomate should know about karaya, a natural gum resin that's available in powder form, disks, or sheets made of karaya and glycerine. Karaya is the most important item in good stoma care. It's the only substance that can be safely applied to an inflamed stoma, tolerate an appliance, and still permit healthy skin to grow. Pure karaya rarely causes allergic reactions, but some preparations with additives do. It is available from many manufacturers or ostomy suppliers. To get an idea of the types of supplies available to ostomy patients, write for the catalogues distributed by these companies: Bruce Medical Supply, 411 Waverly Oaks Rd., Waltham, Mass. 02154; Ostomed Inc., 2715 N. Central, Chicago, Ill. 60639; The Parthenon Co., Inc., 3311 West 2400 South, Salt Lake City, Utah 84119.

If your patient runs out of karaya, here is a temporary karaya substitute: a denture cream called Fasteeth, in which karaya is the primary ingredient.

The enterostomal therapist, physician, or local ostomy association can tell you how to get the appropriate ostomy products for your patient.

Pilonidal Cyst

This procedure involves the removal of a liquid-containing capsule in the middle of the lower back just above the buttocks. Call physician if there are:
• any irregularities at the incision site. Note: It takes four to six weeks for this type of wound to heal completely. There is some chance of recurrence.

Skin Grafts

Grafting is the application of portions of skin to a wound to promote healing, fill in a defect, or replace scar tissue. Call physician in case of:
• fever
• inflammation or discharge at either the recipient or donor areas
• blistering or reddening of graft.

Tonsillectomy and Adenoidectomy

When tonsils and/or adenoids have been removed, call physician if:
• there is fever
• there is increased pain
• patient has difficulty sleeping
• bleeding can be seen in coughing, spitting, or vomitus (may appear like coffee grounds).

8

Home-Care Styles for a Sick Child

There are many variations on the theme of caring for a sick child. Yet, regardless of what your style has been, this chapter can improve it.

The next pages will help you better manage the minor ills of your child—from infant to teenager—at home. Later on you will enter the world of the chronically ill child and learn how to prevent the strains of such care from upsetting family and marital harmony.

Ills That Can Ambush Your Child's Health

In the not-too-distant past many childhood illnesses were dreaded diseases that took thousands of young lives or caused disabling aftereffects. Of course, now there are vaccinations to protect children against diphtheria, measles, mumps, German measles, polio, and whooping cough.

However, there still exist illnesses for which there are no vaccines. Illnesses that still ambush lots of children include scarlet fever, colds, flu, strep throat, and chicken pox.

Let the following guide help you spot fourteen of the most common childhood illnesses early. Here you will learn helpful care tips and when to seek the physician's advice.

Chicken Pox

Chicken pox is one of the most contagious communicable diseases. There is, as yet, no immunization to protect people from getting it. The good news is that in most cases it's a self-limiting disease that runs its course and renders its sufferers immune to future bouts. The bad news is that chicken pox can be very dangerous to children (or other home-care patients) already in weakened conditions from serious illness or chemotherapy.

How can you protect the vulnerable child and other susceptible household members? Spot chicken pox early. Ask your physician for instructions about isolating contagious patients from susceptible ones.

Know the warning signs of chicken pox

Rash is often the first sign. It may start as dark pink, flat spots on the chest or stomach and later spread to the face, arms, and legs. Within hours this develops into blisters containing clear fluid with red borders. The blisters will collapse and turn into scabs. Itching begins on the scalp and spreads to the back of the trunk. Fever and runny nose occur. Sore throat may emerge, especially when sores are in the mouth.

Care tips

Before you give aspirin to reduce fever and/or other discomforts, know that research strongly suggests that aspirin given to children with chicken pox has been linked to Reye's syndrome, a rare children's disease. The syndrome is a life-threatening condition noted by sudden onset of fever and severe headache. It can progress quickly to convulsions and coma. Nearly 30% of its victims die, and some survivors suffer brain damage.

In the past few years several studies have suggested that when aspirin is used to reduce the child's fever from chicken pox (or flu), Reye's syndrome seemed to occur. Let me add there is controversy over this association. Aspirin manufacturers contend that there is no connection between their products and Reye's syndrome. However, a significant number of health organizations and government agencies have issued warnings. Although all the evidence is not in, there is ample reason for concern.

You are best advised to consult your pediatrician before giving your child (up to age eighteen) aspirin for fever in cases of chicken pox (or flu). Your physician can suggest fever-reducing alternatives most appropriate for your child such as acetaminophen or tepid baths.

Ask your child to avoid scratching. If this is impossible, the pediatrician can suggest ways to ease itching such as antihistamines or calamine lotion.

Call physician if treatment does not relieve symptoms or your child experiences:

- high fever
- persistent vomiting
- stuporous behavior
- convulsions.

Colds

Colds and their annoying nasal and throat symptoms strike all children, from infants to teenagers. Many parents automatically ask the physician to prescribe antibiotics to cure their children's colds. The fact is antibiotics can't cure colds, may aggravate your child's symptoms, and in some cases cause a serious allergic reaction.

Know the warning signs of a cold
Runny nose, sneezing, muscle aches, headache, nasal congestion, watery eyes, breathing problems, sore throat, fever, and dry cough are the classic symptoms of a cold.

Care tips
Monitor your child's fever and record on the Home-Health Chart. Consult pediatrician if fever of 101°F. persists more than three days. Provide liquids frequently.

Infants less than six months may benefit from nose drops made of a salt water (saline) solution. Such a solution may be made at home or purchased over the counter at a drugstore. Ask pediatrician for guidance and suggestions for removing mucus from the baby's nose. Nasal syringes may be used to remove mucus. Vaporizers may be considered to ease breathing difficulties.

Children six months and older may be helped by nasal spray decongestants to ease stuffiness. Salt water gargles every two hours may ease sore throat pain in an older child.

Hard candies or cough drops may ease throat discomfort. (Do not give to infants.)

Call physician if your child:
- has a puslike discharge from the nose
- has chest pain or an earache
- seems very ill or displays symptoms for which you are unprepared
- is not better after three days.

Diarrhea

Diarrhea can be caused by many things including viruses, bacteria, emotional upset, food allergies, medication side effects, parasites, and so on. Almost all children experience diarrhea at one time or another. However, there is reason for concern if a child is having one diarrheal stool after another. The reason: Dehydration can occur.

Know the signs of diarrhea
Frequent loose or liquid bowel movements. They may be light brown or green. Diarrhea may appear along with stomach and intestinal infections, colds, and sore throats; stomach cramps may occur.

Care tips
For infants the danger of diarrhea is dehydration (signs: drowsiness, dry mouth, dry coated tongue, lethargy, scanty urine out-

put, fever). Diarrhea problems in infants can usually be corrected with diet changes. Call pediatrician. In older children dehydration is not usually a problem. However, temporary diet changes may be needed to give the intestinal tract a rest. No solid foods or milk for twenty-four hours is often recommended, although plenty of clear liquids should be provided (see Chapter 6). A return to light foods in the next twenty-four hours such as crackers, toast, cereal, and clear liquids may help. On the third day a regular diet may be tried.

Call physician if:
• Your child has abdominal pain *and* vomiting
• Your child has blood in the stool
• Your child is dehydrated (signs indicated above)
• Your child has diarrhea after solid foods and milk have been eliminated from diet
• Your child has a fever of 102°F. for more than 24 hours
• Your child has persistent abdominal pain.

Earache

Earaches are especially common in children. They are most often caused by a bacterial infection.

Know the warning signs of earache
At this point it may be helpful to differentiate between two major causes of earache. One is an infection of the outside ear canal (commonly called swimmer's ear) that may be caused by swimming, foreign bodies, or probing with cotton swabs. Its signs include discharge, ear pain, and sometimes fever. This condition is usually treated with medicated (antibiotic) ear drops prescribed by the doctor.

The second type of infection affects the middle ear and may be the result of a cold or upper respiratory tract infection (sinus infection); it results in an accumulation of fluid or pus in the middle ear (behind the ear drum). Its signs include ear pain, often fever, reduced hearing, and discharge. This type of infection can lead to hearing loss and is usually treated with decongestants and ear drops. In chronic situations the physician may pass a small tube through the ear drum to the middle ear to allow the latter to drain.

Care tips

The pediatrician will probably prescribe medication such as antibiotics and aspirin, or acetaminophen and/or ear drops. Application of heat may ease your child's discomfort. Your child may feel more comfortable if he or she is in a sitting position instead of a lying down position.

Call physician if your child:

- has ear pain
- feels dizzy
- has hearing difficulties
- has fever over 102°F.
- has ear discharge.

Febrile Convulsions

Febrile convulsions are caused by a high fever at the onset of an infection. Generally speaking, these convulsions are not dangerous, nor do they harm children. There are, however, some children who experience complex fever convulsions which can be serious and sometimes cause brain damage. In the event that your child has any signs of convulsions it is essential that you call the physician at once so that a proper medical evaluation can be made.

The tendency toward febrile convulsions runs in families. They most frequently occur in children under the age of three and rarely after age six.

Know the warning signs of febrile convulsions

Your child may have a threshold for convulsions. For example, some kids have seizures at 103°F., some at higher temperatures.

Note the signs: eyes may be fixed or rolling upward; arms, legs, and body may twitch convulsively, nausea, vomiting, unconsciousness.

Care tips
Stay calm. Keep your child from hurting him/herself. If possible place on stomach and turn head to one side to prevent choking on saliva or vomitus. Don't place your fingers, liquids, or medication in your child's mouth. Call physician.

The seizure will usually last several minutes and will stop by the time you reach the doctor. Regardless, it's essential to your child's well-being that the cause of convulsions be pinpointed. Some can be caused by brain infection—a very serious ailment that requires immediate medical treatment. If the doctor is unavailable take your child to the nearest treatment facility.

If the physician is en route to your home, you will want to bring the fever down. Ask him or her for specific instructions. If feasible, the child may be immersed in a tub filled with water below his or her body temperature. (The water should measure between 98°F. and 100°F. See Chapter 4.) Be careful that your child does not get chilled and shiver. Shivering can send fever back up again. Ask physician about using aspirin or acetaminophen.

Fever

Fever is a sign that says the body is fighting an infection or disease.

Know the warning signs of fever
Your child's body will probably be warm to your touch. He or she may appear flushed, perspiring, fatigued; have chills. Take temperature with thermometer (see Chapter 4). Record on Home-Health Chart.

Care tips

Many pediatricians believe that it's not necessary to treat a child's fever with aspirin or acetaminophen until it goes over 102°F. Ask your pediatrician for his or her opinion.

Don't be afraid to bring your child to the pediatrician's office if he or she has a fever. It isn't likely that this will worsen the illness.

See Chapter 4 for suggestions to help you reduce your child's fever. Be sure to offer your child plenty of liquids.

Call the physician if your child:

• develops fever in combination with chronic illness or other serious disease

• develops fever in combination with medical treatment such as chemotherapy or new medication

• is younger than six months and has a fever

• has a low-grade fever for twenty-four hours without other symptoms

• experiences a convulsion

• has a fever over 104°F. without other symptoms.

German Measles

German measles is a common viral disease that causes a rash. It is worth noting that German measles is similar to regular measles. However, the main difference between the two is that regular measles is usually accompanied by intense cold symptoms. German measles sometimes has cold symptoms, but most often they are mild.

One more important point: A pregnant woman without immunity who has been exposed to a child with German measles is at great risk, especially in the first three months of pregnancy. German measles can cause heart disease, blindness, and deafness in the unborn child. Therefore, it is essential that a pregnant woman who has been exposed to German measles call her physician within twenty-four hours for advice.

Know the warning signs of German measles

A small rash, slightly raised spots, low fever, tender and/or swollen glands in the back of the neck, and achiness indicate the presence of this illness. Often the rash does not itch and usually it disappears in three days.

Care tips

Your child's discomforts, such as fever and achiness, may be eased with aspirin or acetaminophen.

Call physician if you are a pregnant woman who has been exposed to German measles who has not been previously immunized.

Measles

This viral disease is known by its rash and cold symptoms.

Know the warning signs of measles

The rash will appear on the third or fourth day following intense cold symptoms such as runny nose, watery eyes, and sensitivity of eyes to light. An initial low fever may rise when the rash appears.

Care tips

Know that this illness can lead to complications. Therefore, it is important to confirm the diagnosis of measles with the physician and to be alert to alarming signs: persistent fever, vomiting, excessive sleepiness, disorientation and/or breathing difficulties.

Because your child's eyes may be sensitive to light, keep his or her room darkened; dark glasses may be tried, too.

Aspirin, acetaminophen, and cold medicines may help to alleviate discomforts.

Call physician if you observe that your child has:
• persistent cough
• breathing difficulties
• earache

- vomiting
- excessive lethargy or sleepiness
- confused behavior.

Mumps

Mumps is a viral illness that causes tenderness and swelling of the salivary glands.

Know the warning signs of mumps
They are indicated by swelling in front of one or both ears, fever, ear pain aggravated by chewing and/or swallowing, and discomfort during chewing or swallowing.

Care tips
Aspirin or acetaminophen can ease unpleasant discomforts. Do not serve sour or highly seasoned foods as they can make your child more uncomfortable.
Call physician if your child experiences:
- sudden headache
- nausea
- vomiting
- excessive drowsiness
- a bad stomach ache or testicular pain and/or tenderness.

Scarlet Fever

This illness is caused by the same bacteria as strep throat. Be aware that scarlet fever can lead to complications in some patients.

Know the warning signs of scarlet fever
These include fever, sore throat, vomiting, rough, red rash that pales for brief moments when pressed with your fingers, swollen glands in the neck.

Care tips

This illness needs medical evaluation and proper management from the pediatrician because of its ability to lead to complications. Most likely he or she will prescribe antibiotics. Aspirin or acetaminophen can reduce other discomforts.

Call physician if you suspect that your child has scarlet fever—even if symptoms seem mild.

Sore Throat

Most sore throats are of little concern. However, they should be watched because in some cases they may be associated with a more significant health problem.

Know the warning signs of sore throat

Suspect sore throat in an infant if he or she refuses to eat; in other children if there is irritability, throat pain, swollen glands, uncomfortable swallowing.

Care tips

Aspirin or acetaminophen can somewhat reduce throat pain. Hard candy, honey, or throat lozenges can also lessen throat discomfort.

Call physician if your child has:
- tenderness and swelling in the neck
- recently been exposed to strep throat
- high fever
- breathing difficulties
- rash
- sore throat persisting more than four days.

Stomach Ache

Here, you should be concerned with any pain in the abdominal area.

Know the warning signs of stomach pain

In infants watch your baby's body language: he or she may tense up, look strained and uncomfortable, draw up knees, be crying and red faced. In all children abdominal pain may be associated with vomiting, diarrhea, nausea, and fever.

Care tips

Provide only clear liquids. Avoid milk and milk products until your child's symptoms disappear.

Heat applied to the stomachs of older children can diminish pain. Use a heating pad, warm wash cloth, or hot water bottle.

Check with physician before giving any medication. Aspirin, for example, may irritate the stomach so acetaminophen may be preferable. Anticramping medication should be given only with physician's consent.

Call physician if your child:
• has stomach pain that persists more than three hours
• has bloody stools
• throws up green vomitus
• appears very ill
• has fever lasting more than twenty-four hours
• has an area that is very sensitive to pressure.

Strep Throat

Strep throat is a highly communicable throat infection.

Know the warning signs of strep throat

These include sore throat, fever, headache, swollen lymph glands, rash (occasionally), abdominal pain, vomiting.

Care tips

Call the physician for proper medical evaluation. He or she can prescribe antibiotics to clear up this illness.

Lessen your child's uncomfortable symptoms with aspirin or

acetaminophen, throat lozenges, honey, hard candy.

Call physician if you have any questions as to the seriousness of your child's throat infection; strep throat can have serious consequences, such as rheumatic fever and kidney problems.

Vomiting

Vomiting accompanies many illnesses and has many causes. In children, it is most commonly caused by viral infections of the stomach and intestines.

Know the signs of vomiting
Vomiting, of course, is obvious, but sometimes food is brought up through the nose.

Care tips
For infants; get immediate medical advice if baby is under six months. Do not give milk. For other children, once vomiting has stopped for several hours offer your child cool, clear liquids frequently. Slowly increase clear liquids, then offer a bland diet (toast, applesauce, Jell-O, etc.). Do not give milk or milk products. After twenty-four hours, offer regular food.

Call physician if:
• your child is excessively sleepy or stuporous
• vomiting persists during a twelve-hour period
• vomiting is accompanied by headache, sleepiness, high fever, breathing difficulties, abdominal pain
• vomitus is green or yellow more than one or two times
• vomiting occurs after recent bout with flu or chicken pox.

Thirst Tempters to Help Your Child Drink Liquids

Your child's illness may require lots of fluids—but getting the youngster to drink them may be a problem. What to do?

Make a list of your child's favorite beverages and the temperatures at which they are most appreciated. (See Chapter 6.)

Offer them in small glasses, if the child is old enough, so that your child feels triumphant when they're empty.

You'll soon discover that liquids become tedious before too long. To combat this, turn liquid drinking into an amusement. For instance, tell the young child to imagine that he or she is a machine that needs fuel to run. Or try colorful straws, uniquely shaped glasses, mugs with favorite movie heroes or cartoon characters. An older child may cooperate if given the task of taking his or her own fluids and keeping a record of them on the Home-Health Chart or similar sheet. Perhaps the youngster can help prepare the beverages. For example, squeezing the fruits for fruit juices, making a cup of tea or clear broth, mixing chocolate or other syrup into milk, adding a dollop of whipped cream from a dispenser, and so on. All should be done under your supervision so that liquids are not forgotten and accidents are avoided.

Other thirst tempters: Saltine crackers, if permitted on your child's diet, can help work up a thirst; ice chips from favorite fruit juices can be sucked to help avoid dehydration when the child refuses to drink. And remember to gently praise your child's efforts. Your warm encouragement and approval may provide just the spur that is needed.

Feeding the Sick Child

Feeding the sick child has been known to frustrate even the most patient parents. Don't panic. Most often this problem can be overcome with some perseverance and imagination.

Obviously, the ill child must eat to maintain weight and strength. If your child refuses food for twenty-four hours or more, consult the physician. Meanwhile, here are some tips that may help you prepare meals your child will accept (also see Chapter 6).

• Many kids detest creamed foods. That nixes casseroles or any dish where the ingredients are combined in a sauce. Solution: Try plain rice or noodles. Consider mixing in hamburger bits or cheese pieces for protein.

• Vegetables turn many children off. Solution: Exchange the

benefit of one vegetable for another fruit or vegetable that has the same nutrients—but more kid-appeal. For example, take broccoli. It's packed with vitamin A—and many children hate it. So try apricots or cantaloupe instead. They're rich in vitamin A and have more appeal for children. (See Chapter 6 for more ideas.)

• Store child-sized portions of your child's favorite dishes in the freezer. Then, if you're serving the family a meal that your youngster rejects, just pop a frozen food into the oven as needed.

• Does your child have a favorite food? One mother told me that her child would only eat hamburgers. She was worried about the nutritional value of a diet based on burgers so she called the pediatrician. The doctor said that it was important that the child "eat something." If it was hamburgers, then so be it. The mother gradually tried to subtly add other foods with the burgers. She covered the patties with cheese, placed them atop rice or noodles, added carrot sticks and other vegetables. If your child has a favorite food, check with the physician to see if a steady diet of it is okay. If it is, serve it as the main dish—and gradually add other foods for more balanced nutrition.

• Serve food in unique ways. Take Popsicle sticks and tooth-picks. Stick them into pieces of fruit, cheese, meat, vegetables. You'll be surprised how a novel approach can tempt a minuscule appetite. Serve cereal in a mug; chicken salad, tuna salad, or cottage cheese in an ice cream cone. A celery stick can be used to hold a cheese spread or chopped salads. Apple slices can be used to hold peanut butter, melted cheese.

Warning: Illness can diminish appetites. Emotional distress, too, can reduce a child's desire for food. Watch your child carefully for emotional causes that may be sabotaging his or her appetite. Questions about this concern should be directed to your physician. Remember, too, not to be overly concerned about a balanced diet if your child is a picky eater. Just offer a variety of foods.

Tips to Meet Your Child's Emotional Needs During Home Care

Take a close look at your sick child. Can you imagine what's going on inside his or her young head? So many possibilities—from worry and frustration to fear and helplessness to scary fantasies and misconceptions. Your child needs lots of love and caring at this time; and there are a few things you can do to help your child feel extra safe and secure:

• Give infants lots of extra snuggling. The closeness and warmth of your body can relieve an unhappy baby who depends on the communication of body contact.

• Help your child feel more secure by responding as soon as possible when he or she calls for you.

• Make time to visit your child's room often. This eases feelings of isolation and reassures the child that he or she has not been forgotten.

• Provide distracting activities (see Chapter 3).

• Tune into your child's words. Younger kids aren't always able to articulate their needs as precisely as adults. Listen carefully to the way your child says something. Watch for body language during conversation. Pick up clues that can reveal your child's inner feelings.

• Encourage your child to talk about his or her feelings. Respond to what you hear with attentiveness and tenderness.

Tantrums

Poor health can make your child cranky. That's normal and to be expected. Sometimes, though, the stresses of illness can transport a child back to an earlier emotional time; a time of greater dependency and less control. This is usual and happens fairly often. You may see it as a temper tantrum, which is best described as kicking, shrieking, foot stomping, and constantly refusing to obey you.

A full-fledged temper tantrum is a frightening sight. Your child may flail about obnoxiously and uncooperatively. Worse yet, in extreme situations the youngster may hold his or her breath, in some cases convulse, and in rare situations lose consciousness. This type of tantrum is most common between the ages of one and three.

Breath holding can be a problem. Because a breath-holder resembles a child experiencing seizures, it's important to differentiate between the two. Here's how to tell them apart.

• Temper tantrums are frequently caused by emotional upset and/or fatigue. Seizures occur suddenly and are often the result of high fevers associated with drowsiness and disturbed consciousness.

• After a temper tantrum your child will seem wide-awake, responsive. The aftermath of a seizure will leave a child sleepy, not alert.

How to Head Off the Tantrum

You know your child and no one else does, so try to zero in on the reason for the difficult mood. Common causes are hunger, fatigue, discomforts of illness, hospitalization, reactions to the word "no," and to overprotectiveness, and attention getting. Once you've figured out the cause try to eliminate it or lessen its effect.

It's worth noting that an ill child may not always understand why he or she must obey certain commands or avoid particular activities. Consequently, your patient may continue to challenge you, doing exactly what you have already said not to do. Saying no all the time may only make matters worse. Instead, try to provide an alternative activity to distract your child's attention.

Confinement can also push some children to the limit. Allow your child to leave the sickroom if the physician permits. The den, living room, or even another bedroom can offer a needed change of scene. One more thing: If your child is confined to the sickroom, consider doing some of your household chores there. It's an easy way to offer companionship while doing tasks such as ironing, sewing, and some aspects of food preparation.

Taking the Sting out of Your Child's Hospital Stay

Five-year-old Douglas needed to have his tonsils out. He was a well-behaved, cooperative boy, so his parents thought the only preparation he needed for the hospital was to be told when the operation was scheduled.

Surgery was the expected success and Douglas was sent home shortly thereafter. After convalescing for a few days it was clear that Douglas had changed. Every night at bedtime he created a commotion. Afraid of the dark and not wanting to be left alone, he screamed and cried. His parents didn't understand why their son had changed.

Recent studies show that for many children a hospital stay can leave emotional scars. For example, studies indicate that children under age five often encounter emotional problems such as a return of bedwetting and anxiousness in the presence of strangers, even after a brief hospitalization. Children five years and older who have been hospitalized for more than a week frequently experience difficulties such as an increase in aggressive behavior and learning problems. Teenagers who have been depressed and commit suicide are more likely to have had a hospital experience earlier in their lives than depressed teenagers who do not.

An important way to diminish the possibility of emotional damage from hospitalization is to prepare your child for the experience.

To begin, your own attitude about your child's impending hospital stay will be relayed to your child regardless of his or her age. The more upset you appear, the more difficult it will be for your child to cope. Clearly, this is a time for you to project support, reassurance, and plenty of love.

Honesty, too, is essential to help enhance your child's trust in you and his or her feeling of security. Your child should be told in language he or she can understand that hospitalization is necessary. Some medical professionals suggest that toddlers be told about three days prior to admission, pre-schoolers about four or five days, school children a week or two before, and adolescents as soon as the hospital stay is scheduled.

What should you tell your child and how should you prepare him or her? Again, this depends on the child's age and the type of procedure entailed. Ask the pediatrician or pediatric nurse for advice to help communicate the need for hospitalization to your child in an appropriate and honest way. Book and patient education materials may help at this time. Turn to medical professionals for book ideas. Also, voluntary health agencies related to your child's illness (American Cancer Society, Spina Bifida Association, etc.) often provide extensive bibliographies and pamphlets targeted to children.

What are the anticipatory feelings of a child in regard to the hospital experience? This, again, depends on the child's age and level of understanding. Most children have rich imaginations and their preconceived visions of the hospital scene may have little to do with the real thing. Furthermore, a child who has already been hospitalized may remember the previous experience as frightening, painful, or lonely and not wish to repeat it.

Here's an idea of some of the anticipatory feelings children in different age groups face.

• A pre-schooler may believe that medical procedures such as surgery or chemotherapy are punishments for being bad, unless reassured that they are needed to help him feel better and get well.

• An elementary school age youngster may grasp the need for surgery but not understand its full meaning. For instance, he or she may think that a surgeon must first remove the legs before taking out an appendix or that when an incision is made all the insides fall out. Clearly, misconceptions must be detected as soon as possible and corrected.

• An upper grade schooler nearing puberty may fear that when his or her parents leave the hospital they will be unable to find their way back. Such insecurities can be more frightening than hospitalization.

• An adolescent trying to seem grown-up may really conceal

strong fears associated with discomfort, separation from parents, and even the possibility of death. Certainly, children should be made to feel that their fears are understood and that they are not alone; that they have the love and support of their families.

Along these lines there has been an increase in the number of pre-hospital programs for children throughout the country. These programs try to allay children's fears by familiarizing them with the hospital environment *before* the stay takes place. Here, children are prepared for medical procedures with explanations by professionals to illuminate their understanding of what to expect. They may include hospital tours, films about treatment and illnesses, and play therapy. Play therapy helps a child express his or her feelings, learn about the condition, act out worries and anxieties, and gain a greater sense of control over his or her life. Many of these programs are geared toward pre-schoolers and elementary-school-age children. In addition, a significant number of programs continue after a child's admission.

There are many ways to address the emotional needs of a child who is about to be hospitalized, no matter what his or her age. Consider these suggestions.

• Ask the pediatrician, pediatric nurse, social worker, or local hospital public relations office to find out if pre-hospital programs are available in your community.

• Contact the voluntary health agency that specializes in your child's illness. Ask if they offer patient education materials that can better your child's understanding of his or her condition and the prescribed medical treatment. Be sure to indicate your child's age and level of schooling.

• In addition to professional advice, help your child prepare for the institutional setting by driving to the hospital so that he or she knows what it looks like. Then drive straight home to reassure your child (especially children under ten) that you know the way.

• Encourage your child to express his or her feelings about the impending hospital experience. For example, a child under five may not articulate his or her emotions in adult terms, but you can learn a great deal by watching closely as he or she plays. Toys, stuffed animals, and fantasies may be the vehicles your child uses to express inner thoughts and ideas. Games involving a newly wounded stuffed animal, for instance, suggest that your child may be anxious about his or her own health. If your child is of school age, try to detect if he or she is harboring misunderstandings about planned medical procedures. Gently correct wrong ideas if they exist. An adolescent may need you to provide a caring and accepting ear. Surely some adolescents don't want to be thought of as "children" and may hold in their true feelings. Watch for changes in appetite, behavior, sleep patterns, and body language that can signal emotional distress.

• Stay with your child during medical procedures whenever possible. Some children, especially pre-schoolers, may find separation from parents more frightening than the medical treatment. In such cases, spend the night in the hospital room with your child.

• Insist on being present during diagnostic test such as X rays, intravenous insertions, etc. Be as close by as possible when your child receives an anesthetic. Of course, there are times when your presence is inappropriate. You know your child better than anyone, so try to tune into his or her emotional needs. Older children and younger children alike may need the security of a parent who is close by to lend a familiar voice and loving words. Remember, though, that some children may want to be independent or simply want their privacy. Be sensitive to such needs and follow your instincts.

When Your Child Is Chronically Ill

The child who is chronically ill has very special health and emotional needs. The second half of this chapter will show you how to manage many of the important tasks facing you and your child at this time.

How to Increase the Benefits
of Your Child's Radiation Therapy

In Chapter 3 you learned about radiation therapy for adults. Here are some additional considerations for children.

If radiation therapy is prescribed for your child it is critical that he or she cooperate with medical technicians during the procedure to receive optimum benefit. Radiation therapy may be performed while your child is hospitalized on an out-patient basis.

Encouraging your child to cooperate with medical personnel is essential. This is rarely a problem for older children. Unfortunately, the wiggling and squirming of toddlers and pre-schoolers may interfere with proper treatment. To avoid this, prepare your young one for treatments by practicing them at home. Try this: Use a table, or if the child is bedridden the bed will do. What is your goal? To urge your child to stay still and immobilized for longer and longer periods of time. Add authenticity by using a camera in place of the radiation machine. Ask your child to hold still and then "take a picture." Let your child know that this is practice for the real radiation treatment in the hospital and that it won't hurt a bit.

After-care for radiation therapy: Again, see Chapter 3 for a detailed description of aftereffects. Add to them the following for children: If diarrhea occurs, keep child's perianal area clean to prevent inflammation and infection. If hair loss occurs keep your child's head protected in cold weather to prevent heat loss. Ask the physician for additional advice. Call physician if nausea and vomiting persist, signs of dehydration appear, bleeding develops, oral and rectal ulcers occur; if there is coughing, chest pain, headache, edema, malaise.

Your Child and Chemotherapy

Although Chapter 3 deals with this subject, there are some additional concerns regarding children and chemotherapy.

Chemotherapy affects the bone marrow, and this can drain the body's ability to fight infection. Children may become susceptible to certain illnesses to which adults already have immunity. One potentially dangerous illness is chicken pox (discussed earlier in this chapter). A child who comes down with a secondary infection while already in a weakened state is in a potentially serious position. The bottom line: Children undergoing chemotherapy always should be isolated from others who are ill. Consult physician for guidance.

Know, too, that chemotherapy can cause wounds and injuries to take a longer time to heal. So protect your child by keeping the home safe and preventing accidents. Remove low tables with sharp edges, keep floors uncluttered to prevent falls, forbid contact sports and rough games.

One more thing: Watch for ulcers and infections that may appear on mucous membranes. The most common is called oral candidiasis. You can spot it by looking for white patches that may appear inside your child's mouth. Make sure your patient follows good oral hygiene as a further safeguard (see Chapter 3).

Home Care and the Chronically Ill Child

Chronic illness—that's the phrase used for a long-term disorder that can be debilitating, deteriorating, and sometimes fatal. The list is a long one, from cancer and cerebral palsy, to asthma and cystic fibrosis, from heart disease and spina bifida to diabetes and kidney disease—and many more, each with its own unique set of problems.

You may be filled with many questions and fears if the doctor says that your child has a chronic illness. How will the illness change my child's life? Are the prescribed medications or treatments painful or dangerous? Is the illness more serious than the doctor said? Is it hereditary?

To cope with your questions and concerns, learn everything you can about your child's ailment and its treatment. Ask your physician to clarify anything you don't understand. If he or she is not responsive to your questions, or if you are still confused about your child's condition, ask to be referred to another, more communicative physician.

Chances are there's a voluntary health organization that supplies information about your child's illness. Phone or write for their publication lists. Moreover, there are support and self-help groups in many communities to help you and your child manage the repercussions of the chronic condition (see Chapter 14 for addresses and/or check your telephone directory under the listing of the illness, "Diabetes," "Cancer," "Heart," etc.).

Ignorance is not the only thing that sabotages successful home care for chronic illnesses. You may also be setting emotional traps for yourself along the way. Guilt is the biggest. You love your child and it may be heartbreaking for you to watch as he or she is undermined by illness. Do you replay any of the following phrases in your mind? *If only I had paid more attention to my son's complaints. Did my daughter inherit her illness from me? Why wasn't I a better mother?* These are common refrains. Try not to let them get the best of you.

When my father was ill I worried that I was in some way responsible. The guilt shadowed me for some time. Eventually, I discussed my feelings with my brother—and learned that he was experiencing the same emotions.

You, too, may find comfort by sharing your thoughts and anxieties with your spouse, friends, and/or close relatives. If that isn't possible for you, or if you don't find relief, turn to your medical advisor, nurse, or social worker for more professional counseling.

There's another emotional trap to beware of—overprotecting your child. It's natural to want to shield your loved one from activities and situations you think will aggravate the chronic illness. But too much overprotectiveness can do more harm than good. It can deny a child the freedom to explore his or her potential. It sometimes can set the young one apart from peers. Moreover, it can create an overdependent child—and the youngster can grow into an overdependent adult.

Ask the physician to list your child's limitations. Then encourage your child to reach for his or her maximum potential. Most hampered children need encouragement to do tasks on their own. Growth experiences—and the opportunity to rise past disabilities—are denied the overprotected child. Encourage small tasks first, so once they're mastered your child will feel inspired to go on.

How to Sharpen Your Insight into the Chronically Ill Child

Because each child has his or her own set of unique emotional and physical needs, it is wise that you discuss your child's particular situation with medical professionals. Use the following as a supplement to the information you receive.

Your Chronically Ill Baby

If your child has been diagnosed as having a chronic illness you may be faced with one of the most difficult emotional experiences in home care for children. Shocked and worried about your baby, you may wonder how you will find the strength to provide care. And you may be afraid to get emotionally close to your baby. Indeed, this may be your way of safeguarding yourself if you fear he or she may die.

Unlike healthy babies, a very ill one may fill you with intense disappointment. This is sharpened when your child looks sickly, has abnormalities, or appears lifeless. Rather than being wide-eyed and aglow, the sick infant may seem pitiful, perhaps even repulsive to you or your mate.

If these feelings seem at all familiar, rest assured that they are quite normal. However, it is essential that you get past your personal pain because your baby needs you. Your child, helpless and ill, needs all the love, caring, and bodily contact you can give to help maintain health and develop. Your cuddling, talking, and nurturing will stimulate the child, boosting the baby's sense of security and trust so crucial in the healing process.

How can you meet your baby's needs in the midst of your own worry and grief? Zero in on what may be shaking your care-confidence. Discuss these problems with the physician or other pediatric professional. Perhaps you feel emotionally distanced from your child because he or she does not resemble the cooing, robust infant you expected. Maybe home treatments seem complicated and forbidding, and you are afraid to tackle them. These are normal situations that can certainly be managed with the proper professional guidance.

How to Recapture Your Care-Giving Confidence

Start by recognizing that your feelings of grief, sadness, disappointment, failure, repulsion, and/or anxiety are not abnormal. Rest assured that they can frequently be managed and with help and in time overcome. This, with counseling from the pediatrician, pediatric nurse, or child psychologist or psychiatrist. Express your feelings to your mate, relatives, and/or trusted friends. Your ability to help your child is not increased by denying your emotions. It is, however, enhanced by a mature acceptance of the situation, seeking help if needed, and reaching out to give the baby the love and care it deserves.

Certainly, it may not be easy to provide home care for a chronically ill infant and cope with your emotional responses as well as your other family obligations. Therefore, consider the help of friends, relatives, or neighbors to pitch in to lessen your burden of responsibility. Medical professionals such as visiting nurses or other home-care helpers, as well as baby sitters and volunteers from community and religious organizations, can all provide assistance.

One more thing: Although your baby may not be as responsive as a healthy one, he or she needs as much attention, stimulation, and bodily contact as a well one. When you find it overwhelming to give as much as the baby needs, think of "stand-ins" that can help while you take time for yourself. The voice of a radio, television, record or video tape can be turned on at a comfortable level near the baby. The sounds and visuals can periodically rouse the child when you cannot be there. Older children, your mate, and relatives can be directed to tenderly massage the baby's hands, feet, and/or limbs. (Be sure to check with the physician about the amount of activity and movement that is needed for your child. Adhere to prescribed exercises.) Photographs or mobiles may be placed in sight of the baby. The baby's crib may be moved into the midst of family activity (discussions, game playing, meals, television watching). Think of alternatives to your presence when you are unable to give the frequent human contact your child needs.

The Chronically Ill Child, Ages Three to Five

Here is a child who is gaining a stronger sense of him- or herself every day. He or she is mastering new skills, making new discoveries. It becomes increasingly more important for the young child to become more assertive, more able to do things on his or her own. Without a doubt illness can wreak havoc with your child's needs for more independence and assertiveness. Chronic illness may mean your child depends on you to help him or her eat, dress, use the bathroom—skills he or she may have already learned to do alone.

To counteract regression, help your child by allowing him or her as much responsibility as the illness permits. Turn to the pediatrician or nurse to suggest ways your patient can help with treatments, administering medication and other care tasks, ways to underscore his or her emerging sense of self.

Your young patient's needs for more freedom may also make some aspects of home care problematic if he or she challenges you by being uncooperative during treatment, refuses to do prescribed exercises, or rejects medication and food. You may find yourself furious at your child's behavior, yet reluctant to reprimand because he or she is ill. Or your anger may build up, pushing you close to and sometimes dangerously past your emotional limits. Here are two possible solutions: Give your child as much control over care tasks as he or she is capable of. Discuss persistent problems with medical professionals to gain suitable insights.

Remember, too, that this is the age when your child is becoming increasingly aware of his or her body and the image it projects. Clearly, any illness that causes disability, deformity, or unattractive symptoms can undermine your child's feelings of confidence and worth. Once again you can be supportive by encouraging (not pushing!) your patient to ventilate his or her feelings about the visible signs of the illness. Create an atmosphere of acceptance and caring. Help your child focus on his or her positive attributes.

Your child will also get a stronger feeling of control and participation during home care if given accurate information about his or her condition. Patient education materials geared toward very young children can help your child better understand the condition and its treatment. If you see that your child has misconceptions replace them with honest and easy-to-understand explanations. Medical professionals can offer advice regarding this problem.

Chronic Illness in Children Five to Eleven Years Old

Many children at this age want to be like their peers. However, chronic illness may make your child feel quite different from other children of the same age. For example, he or she may look different because of the illness or because of the side effects of the treatments. Your child may be separated from the group if he or she must avoid rambunctious play activities. Possibly your youngster must follow a restricted diet or take medication according to a rigid schedule. Each situation can act to separate your child from the group, ultimately causing much distress.

This is a rough situation. One of the best ways you can come to your youngster's aid is by helping him or her to accept the illness. Your child may need to develop coping skills that make it easier to field the questions and ridicule that may go on in the company of other children. The pediatrician, nurse, or child psychologist may be helpful here. Meet with your child's teacher and/or principal to discuss the illness and special care that may be needed during school hours. Be sure that you are made aware of emotional and physical problems as they arise, so they can receive your prompt attention.

As with other children, your school-age child will benefit if he or she is allowed to help administer treatments and assume responsibility for care tasks. This is especially valuable when treatments become an integral part of your child's life, as in the case of injections for a diabetic. Prepare your patient for possible discomforts, side effects, and reactions that may result from the treatments. If treatment changes in some way (a new prescription is needed, dosage is increased or diminished) tell your child why. If you don't, he or she may imagine that change is a negative sign concerning the illness.

The Chronically Ill Adolescent

Of course, an adolescent is not yet an adult, and so may benefit from some of the guidelines given in the preceding sections on younger children. Beyond that, remember that your adolescent is approaching or is in the middle of great emotional and physical changes. A chronic illness only adds to the changes with which your child must cope. His or her need for independence and acceptance is greater than ever. Body image, too, becomes an exceedingly sensitive area as adolescence is the age of sexual maturing and, ideally, great spurts of physical and emotional growth.

It is extremely important that you know what role, if any, your patient's condition will play during the physical, emotional, and sexual maturation processes of puberty. Will it, for instance, affect growth, sexual development, menstruation, ejaculation? Demand specific information from the physician. Learn as much as you can about the illness's effect on an adolescent by talking to other medical professionals and reading patient education materials.

If, indeed, the illness inhibits growth and development in some way, you will need professional guidance to help you relay this news to your child in the most understanding, supportive, and clear manner possible.

Remember, too, that your adolescent youngster needs the acceptance of his or her peers. An illness that has gone on for a long time may already have weaved its way into the fabric of peer acceptance. But one of recent onset may create new problems for your child. He or she may need to develop coping skills to field explanations when others are inquisitive or mocking.

On the other hand, your child may not want others to know about his or her condition. This is a reasonable choice as long as a denial of the illness does not interfere with your youngster's treatment or progress. You can help your child by creating a cover story that enables the youngster to explain things to others in a way he or she finds comfortable. Of course, it may be important for teachers to know about your child's situation, but in some cases confidentiality is important. Get professional advice. Notify school officials when it is necessary to increase support for your child.

One more thing: Your adolescent is likely to have a strong need to communicate thoughts and feelings at this time. With so many concerns preoccupying the child (appearance, dating, repercussions of illness, sex, success at school) the need for self-expression and sharing feelings may be urgent. Consider the possibility of private counseling. The pediatrician can offer recommendations here for the appropriate child psychologist, psychiatrist, or psychiatric social worker.

Self-help groups, too, can prove invaluable. In such meetings your child can share feelings with other people who have the same illness. (See Chapter 2 for the National Self-Help Clearinghouse, call the voluntary health agency related to your child's illness, or ask the pediatrician for referrals.)

Home-Care Treatments for Your Child

Many ill children, from infants to adolescents, will need home treatments such as medication, injections, physical therapies, respiratory therapies, and special diets.

Although you know that prescribed treatments are meant to help your child, you may dread administering them. After all, every pill or special exercise is a reminder that your child is ill. And some treatments are just plain uncomfortable for the child. Add to this the times your patient will reject or complain about a procedure, your own insecurity about administering the treatment effectively—and you may end up with tensions galore and a potentially serious predicament: Postponing or forgetting about treatment altogether.

Treatments are prescribed to maintain or improve health. Postponing or avoiding them may be doing your child more harm than good. If you have been putting off treatments, giving them haphazardly, or are overanxious when administering them, try to determine the reason for your apprehension.

One mother, for example, was afraid to give her baby daughter injections, so she stopped. Naturally, she realized that something had to be done. She asked herself, Why am I afraid? Very quickly she knew that every time she gave a treatment the child cried. The mother consulted the pediatrician and he suggested that a visiting nurse supervise the injections until the mother's confidence was restored.

Home care for your chronically ill child will be easier if you feel positive about what you are doing. If you remain nervous, your child may sense it and become even more uncooperative.

How to Prepare for Home-Care Treatments

- Preplan a precise schedule—and stick to it.
- Gather together all the equipment you'll need. Then proceed with the treatment.

• Try not to pull your child away from a favorite activity to give a treatment.

• Perform the procedure in a quiet, private place with no distractions.

• Consider playing some calm music to create a serene mood.

• Urge your mate or nearest relative to participate in treatment whenever possible.

• Encourage your child, if possible, to assume some responsibility during treatment. For example if you must give an oral medication, ask your child to pick a beverage to wash it down. If your child is very young, try "giving the treatment" first to a favorite stuffed animal, then to the child.

Warning! Chronic Illness Can Strain Your Marriage

Children feel more safe and secure when they sense that their parents' relationship is a stable one. A strong foundation of family support can help a child muster the courage and strength needed to cope with the effects of illness. Trouble is, it is often chronic illness itself that can shake the supports of even the best marriages.

Studies show that during home care for a chronically ill child, emotional distance can develop between the parents. And the more this gap is allowed to widen, the greater the increase of marital tensions and the risk of divorce. Take the experience of the Smiths, a hypothetical couple based on several real examples.

Jack Smith had been a very involved father. But when his daughter Linda developed leukemia his parenting role went haywire. Jack was a salesman and he had to work extra hours to make the money needed to pay mounting medical bills. The more he worked, the more distanced he felt from the home scene, his child, and his wife, Cathy. While he was feeling helpless and concerned, Cathy had her own set of frustrations. She had the consolation of being directly involved in her child's care, but the burden of most of the nursing tasks fell on her shoulders. She started to resent Jack for being away so much. And Jack continued to work even harder because it seemed to be the only way he could contribute to his daughter's care. Gradually, and insidiously, the distance between the Smiths increased. And so did their marital troubles.

Couples who communicate well with each other, who detect difficulties and deal with them as they arise, are likely to manage the stresses of home care. There are, however, no rules. And the Smiths' troubles are only one example of those that can develop between the parents of a chronically ill child.

My advice: If you sense trouble, discuss it with your partner as soon as possible. If you cannot, seek professional help. Consult your physician, nurse, social worker, or a family therapist for advice. There are also support groups for parents of the chronically ill child. Locate one in your community.

Here are some warning signs to let you know when home-care stresses are affecting your marriage:
- burden of care is falling on one parent
- guilt is overwhelming
- lack of interest in sex
- one partner's sexual interest increases in reaction to the child's illness while the other partner's decreases
- more frequent "blaming" discussions.

What You Should Know About Depression and the Chronically Ill Child

Chronic illness is a constant stress that can wear down your child. It is not a temporary ailment, but a long-lasting one that can indelibly alter your child's life and relationships. It can challenge your child's spirit, and at times whittle it away.

There is nothing mysterious or surprising about the fact that chronic illness can depress a child. The trouble is that mind and body are so integrated that depression can undermine health and health maintenance. How? Depression brings with it symptoms that act to defeat healing and recovery. Loss of appetite, lethargy, and sleeping difficulties, for instance, can drain a child's energies and make the battles of chronic illness tough to fight.

Therefore, spot the signs of depression early and deal with them before they pose a serious threat to your child's emotional and physical health.

Telltale Signs

If any of the following persist, there is serious cause for alarm. Call physician immediately for guidance if your child:
• has poor sleeping habits
• sleeps too much
• shows poor appetite and weight loss
• has difficulty getting along with others (aggressive, hostile behavior)
• says he/she feels ugly, stupid, etc., not like other kids
• shows sadness and weepiness
• has school difficulties—poor memory and concentration, lower grades, resists going to school.

What Triggers Depression?

This, of course depends on the illness and the child. Some children may mourn when the illness prevents them from doing things other kids can do. A boy confined to a wheelchair may be demoralized because he can't run around like other boys his age. A girl with diabetes may worry that she's different from other girls because she must give herself injections and only eat certain foods.

Depression can also appear in the child who feels responsible for his or her illness and its effect on the family. Parents sometimes unwittingly blame the child. *"If you had done exactly what I told you to do you wouldn't have gotten sick."* In turn the child lives with the burden that he or she is at fault. And every time the illness rears its debilitating head the child only feels more helpless.

When a child cannot master certain activities, low moods and sadness can result. The handicap itself becomes a reminder that it has to be overcome.

How Can You Help?

• Youngsters can lose perspective when they only see their world in terms of their own limitations and defects. Learn the latest techniques available to help your child and his or her particular illness. Remarkable strides can be made when individuals face challenges rather than withdraw from them. Provide the concern, encouragement, and love to help your child discover his or her best potential.

• Be realistic about the meaning of your child's illness. Expecting your child to be normal when that is impossible places a heavy burden on the child, which can feed frustration and depression. Your reaction to the illness will affect how your child perceives it and adapts—or fails to adapt—to it.

• Encourage your child to express his or her feelings.

Turn That Sickroom into a Schoolroom

You will want to be sure that your child does not fall too far behind with his or her schoolwork. This, of course, is a real possibility when your child is at home with a long-term illness, or when schooling is interrupted because of repeated visits to the hospital or other treatment facility.

Your child's teacher may be able to help you work out a suitable program. Tutoring may be recommended, or perhaps a special home-study program.

If your child is a college student, there are alternatives, too. Some colleges have special programs for the chronically ill or disabled. As a college professor I have taught students who took my classes from home. They had a phone device that allowed them to listen to a class—and participate via a two-way hookup.

In addition, many urban universities offer television courses for credit.

For more information about education alternatives, write Higher Education and the Handicapped, 1 DuPont Circle, Washington, D.C. 20036 (offers a clearinghouse of information on post-secondary education for the handicapped and disabled); National Home-Study Council, 1601 18 St., N.W., Washington, D.C. 20009 (provides clearinghouse of information on nationwide home-study programs); Council of Better Business Bureaus, 1515 Wilson Blvd., Arlington, Va. 22209. (Ask for their booklet that can help you select a quality home-study program.)

9

Sexuality
and Home Care

For many men and women sex is one of life's most pleasurable experiences: an exquisite communication shared by lovers; a private sensual delight that recharges the body and the spirit.

Unfortunately, illness can send a person's sexuality into a tailspin. Not surprisingly, any illness that brings weakness, fever, fatigue, pain, nausea, dizziness, paralysis, or breathing difficulties can cause sexual problems. So, too, can changes in body image after surgery or accident, spinal cord injury, chronic illness, and mental illness.

If you or your lover is experiencing sexual changes during or after illness you may be wondering what to do. Persistent problems are best taken to your physician or a qualified sex therapist— but more on that later. Meanwhile, let me suggest some topics for you to consider to help clarify your understanding of your partner's situation:

• What is the effect of your loved one's illness on his or her sexual style? Much depends on the nature of his or her condition and sexual style before taking ill. Ask the physician to explain exactly how your partner's condition will affect his or her sex life. Get plenty of information by consulting medical professionals and reading patient education materials. Demand answers to these questions: Does illness pose any sexual limitations? Are there specific sexual techniques or positions that can be tried to lessen dangers or discomforts? Where can you go for sexual counseling, if necessary?

• Is your loved one undermining his or her sexual potential? People often have insufficient information and wrongly assume that sexual activity will interfere with recovery or worsen symptoms. Yes, there are many times when sexual intercourse should be postponed to allow your partner to recover adequately. The physician can tell you when you may resume intercourse. Only rare situations demand that all forms of sexual pleasure be abstained from altogether.

Remember, too, that although sexual intercourse may have to be postponed, there are many sexual avenues still open. Indeed, for the great majority of people, holding, cuddling, kissing, and stroking need not be postponed.

• Is your loved one preoccupied with statistics that indicate sexual function will be limited because of his or her condition? As one certified sex counselor told me, "People shouldn't be deterred by numbers. Each case is different." Remember, statistics offer professionals broad guidelines. For some people who see tham as gospel, percentages can become self-fulfilling prophecies.

• Are you and your loved one realistic about his or her sexual abilities and interests? Certainly, an elderly person who has been ill will not regain the sexual drive of youth after recovery. By the same token, a person who had little interest in sex before illness should not be expected to do a sexual about-face once recovered—unless the ailment caused the problem. Some medications that may be essential to maintain your partner's health may also play a role in your partner's sexual difficulties (antihypertensives, etc.). Sometimes different medications can be tried to alleviate the problem. Occasionally there are no ready alternatives. Furthermore, there are some illnesses that have a direct effect on sexual functioning. The overwhelming majority of these individuals can become reacquainted with their sexual potential. But some readjustments for both partners may be necessary. Sexual counseling can be extremely beneficial here.

• Does the physician diminish your loved one's hopes about sex? There are no hopeless situations. For some people changes may be profound, but everyone is capable of receiving sexual pleasure or giving it in some fashion. It is important to note that there are some physicians who are unable to give educated sexual advice because they are embarrassed by sexual topics or they are not knowledgeable about available alternatives. If you suspect that either is the case with your doctor, consider consulting professionals who specialize in sex counseling for the ill or injured person. See the list of human sexuality programs and other resources that appear later in this chapter.

Does Your Partner (or You) Have Sexual Myopia?

That means a *limited vision of sexuality*. It's a condition that strikes when people see sex only in terms of sexual intercourse.

Sexual myopia was best described to me by a certified sex counselor whose clients are disabled or ill. "People must try to be positive," she said. "Sometimes sex is not the same as it was before their illness. But it is possible to receive pleasure. It is possible to try new things. People may have altered abilities after a disabling illness. This does not mean that they are dysfunctional."

To be sure, it may be difficult for you and your loved one to make changes in your sexual life. But changes can also be viewed as exciting. This may be a time when you and your partner can learn to communicate better, or learn to try things that you have never tried before.

My message is a simple one: Human sexuality involves all the feelings we have as men and women. It's the way we dress, the height of a heel, the way we carry on a conversation. It's the seductive sparkle in someone's eyes, the texture of the skin. Simply being alive is sexual.

People who limit their vision of sexuality only to intercourse deny themselves the other sensual riches and joys the body has to offer. The secret of satisfying lovemaking is not confined to the sex organs. It is the excitement of all the senses and the comfort of sharing ecstatic sensations with a caring and understanding lover.

When Illness Triggers Desire

The depression that may come during illness obviously can dampen the ardor and responsiveness of many affected persons. But there are some people, albeit a small minority, in whom depression is expressed differently. They display an upswing in mood and an increased sexual interest.

For example, one woman who had a mastectomy developed a compulsive need for sex. A man who was terminally ill insisted that his wife masturbate him—despite the fact that he was very ill and had difficulty moving.

If your patient responds to illness with an increased interest in sex, it may come from denial, a strong protest against the illness. He or she may want to deny the loss of a body part, or deny the overwhelming sense of doom that can come with a very serious condition. For some, hypersexuality is a reaffirmation of being alive.

How to Give Your Loved One Sexual Support

Your loved one may be dealing with a host of emotions and, possibly, some sexual difficulties. During this time your partner will need your gentle support and understanding. The more you know about the effect of illness on his or her sexuality, the more insight you will have to handle the situation.

Here are some suggestions that may be helpful to you and your partner.

• If sexual intercourse must be postponed for a short while (or indefinitely), rediscover the wonder of touching. (See Chapter 3.) Massage can be a relaxing experience. It can also be transformed into an erotic one. Books on the subject, especially illustrated ones, can provide inspiration. Hugging, too, is a comforting contact. One good thing about hugging—you almost always get one when you give one.

• If you are having difficulty keeping romance alive in your relationship because as care giver your role has become nurturing and maternal, know that this is not unusual. It may be difficult for you to make the transition from "home nurse" to sexual partner. One way to deal with this: Encourage your patient to be as independent as possible. For example, some care givers find it difficult to feel sexy when only hours before they were administering a bedpan, or managing catheter equipment, or feeding their loved one. It may therefore be helpful to ask or hire others to assist you with certain areas of personal care.

• If you are afraid of hurting your partner during sex it is important that you fully understand your patient's condition so that you know if there are any limitations to be heeded—or if you are unnecessarily anxious. Some care givers fear that love-making can bring on another heart attack or stroke; or that if the patient is not completely recovered, sex is wrong. These notions can cause trouble when they are unfounded. Be totally informed!

• If your partner would benefit from more intense stimulation than would normally be received during intercourse, consider purchasing a vibrator. You may never have thought of using one before illness. Now is the chance to experiment with a new idea. As one sex counselor said, "If it works, terrific. If not, it was only an experiment." Vibrators may be purchased at some pharmacies, through magazines and some special catalogues.

• If your loved one's illness or disability makes disrobing difficult, he or she may need your help. Don't allow disrobing to remind you of your partner's limitations. Instead, work undressing into your sexual activity.

• If your loved one has a motor loss or loss of sensation (caused by stroke, injuries, etc.), you may not know what feels good to him or her. Indeed, your partner's abilities may be altered. This does not mean that he or she cannot enjoy sexual activity. Experiment with your partner so that you will learn which caresses are or are not appreciated. Do not ignore the disabled side or body part. Your accepting touches and kisses can do much for your lover's self-esteem. If communication between you and your lover is difficult at this time, consider the guidance of a sex counselor.

• If you would like to add something new to your sexual repertoire, try doing something that had been postponed or rejected because of your partner's illness. Now that he or she has improved or is well again, these activities may be appropriate to try. For example, certain sexual positions that were impossible during illness may be possible now.

Drugs Can Be Sexual Saboteurs

Did you know that some drugs have side effects that can cause sexual problems? That's why it's important to rule out your loved one's medication as sexual saboteur. The physician can help you. Or you can look up the medication's side effects in the *Physician's Desk Reference* or the *United States Pharmacopeia/Dispensing Information (USP/DI)* (see Chapter 3). Certain drugs have been known to cause loss of sexual interest in both men and women. Others have resulted in erectile problems and ejaculatory difficulties for men, and diminished lubrication and orgasm difficulties for women.

I offer the following list of such drugs as a reference to you. Some drugs under these categories have undermined sexual functioning in certain patients:

anticoagulants
antihypertensives
diuretics
antipsychotics
antidepressants
MAO Inhibitors
anticholinergics

antihistimes
anxiolytics, sedatives, and
hypnotics
amphetamines
steroids
antispasmodics
cytotoxics
ganglionic blockers

Note: There are some medications that increase sexual desire in susceptible people. L-Dopa, a drug used for Parkinson's disease, has been known to have this effect in certain people. Of course, some drugs may appear to do this because they alleviate symptoms that had inhibited sexual functioning.

Where to Get Help

As I mentioned earlier, the physician is the professional to speak to for advice and guidance. But many doctors are either uninformed about or reluctant to discuss sex problems. If your doctor is unable to answer your questions or does not have the expertise to help you with your problems, there are alternatives. You may find it helpful to turn to your gynecologist or urologist. Beyond these possibilities consider a certified sex counselor or therapist. To locate one, call a social worker affiliated with a major medical center (a university teaching hospital, for example) in your area. Ask the social worker for the names of professionals who specialize in the sexuality of the disabled or ill. It is essential that when seeking the help of a sex counselor or therapist you consult someone who is *certified*. One organization that lists certified professionals is The American Association of Sex Educators, Counselors, and Therapists. Write for the *National Register* ($5) for a comprehensive listing of therapists and counselors throughout the country. Send to AASECT, 2000 N St., N.E., Washington, D.C. 20036. (Of course, AASECT does not list *all* qualified professionals.)

Other alternatives: Consult the Department of Psychiatry at a nearby medical school for referrals; contact the nearest Rehabilitation Center associated with a major hospital and ask to speak to the professional who specializes in the sexuality of the disabled. The professional you choose should be experienced with individuals whose illness or disability may be affecting their sexuality. Or you may want to contact one of the sexuality programs offered at a major hospital or university in your community. Here is a partial listing of such programs.

ARIZONA
University of Arizona
  College of Medicine
Sexual Problems and
  Evaluation Clinic
1501 North Campbell Ave.
Tucson, Ariz. 85724

CALIFORNIA
University of California at
  Los Angeles
Human Sexuality Program
Neuropsychiatric Institute
760 Westwood Plaza—Box 4
Los Angeles, Calif. 90024

UNIVERSITY OF CALIFORNIA
School of Medicine at
  San Francisco
Department of
  Psychiatry
Human Sexuality
  Program
400 Parnassus A841
San Francisco, Calif. 94143

CONNECTICUT
University of Connecticut
  Health Center
Department of Psychiatry
Sexual Education and
  Treatment Service
263 Farmington Ave.
Farmington, Conn. 06032

ILLINOIS
Southern Illinois University
  School of Medicine
Department of
  Obstetrics/Gynecology
P.O. Box 3926
Springfield, Ill. 62708

MARYLAND
The Johns Hopkins
  Hospital
Sexual Behaviors
  Consultation Unit
Meyer 101
600 N. Wolfe St.
Baltimore, Md. 21205

MASSACHUSETTS
New England Male
  Reproductive Center of
  University Hospital
720 Harrison Ave.
Suite 606
Boston, Mass. 02118

MINNESOTA
University of Minnesota
  Medical School
Department of Family
  Practice and Community
  Health
Program in Human Sexuality
2630 University Ave., S.E.
Minneapolis, Minn. 55414

NEW YORK
Mount Sinai Medical Center
Department of Psychiatry
Human Sexuality Program
19 E. 98th St.—Rm. 9A
New York, N.Y. 10029

To locate the nearest sexuality clinic that specializes in your patient's type of concern write to Stanley Ducharme, PhD., c/o National Task Force on Sexuality and Disability, University Hospital, 75 E. Newton St., Boston, Mass. 02118.

Additional sources of information include the following.

SIECUS
(Sex Information & Education Council of the U.S.)
80 Fifth Avenue
New York, N.Y. 10011

They publish one of the most comprehensive lists available for consumers that includes a listing of more than a hundred books, periodicals, and organizations relating to sexuality and illness topics. Send $1 and a stamped, self-addressed business-size envelope. Ask for the list called Sexuality and the Disabled.

Human Sciences Press
72 Fifth Ave.
New York, N.Y. 10011

Write for their publication list concerning sexuality and the disabled. Among their titles is *Family Planning and Sexuality Concerns of the Physically Disabled Woman* ($2.50).

Other books you may consider are these.

Sexuality Options for Paraplegics and Quadriplegics, by T.O. Mooney, T.M. Cole, and R.A. Chilgren, Little, Brown & Co., Boston, 1975.

Sexual Consequences of Disability, by Alex Comfort, Philadelphia: George F. Stickley, Co., 1978.

Sexuality and Physical Disability, Personal Perspectives, edited by David and Susan Knight, St. Louis: C.V. Mosby Co., 1981.

Who Cares? A Handbook on Sex Education and Counseling Services for Disabled People, issued by Sex and Disability Project, George Washington University, Washington, D.C., 1979. This publication lists many resources, including a comprehensive listing of sexuality clinics at hospitals and universities throughout the country.

The Intelligent Person's Guide to Illness and Sexuality

The rest of this chapter is a miniguide devoted to certain illnesses that can cause performance anxieties as well as changes in sexual interest and functioning. It is my hope that some of your questions will be answered and that you can put the suggestions for alleviating difficulties to good use.

Important: These pages should be used as a guideline only. Each patient's case is unique and deserves evaluation and treatment by a competent medical professional.

Arthritis

Common concerns

Some people worry that the symptoms of arthritis (limited motion, pain involving the hips, back, and/or knees) can affect sexual functioning. This is a natural concern. Indeed, pain in the joints not specifically involved in sexual activity can detract from pleasure. Your lover may worry that he or she cannot meet your expectations and needs.

Furthermore, some people develop a negative view of themselves because of the physical changes that may have resulted from their arthritis. Your loved one may feel unattractive or undesirable—and withdraw from sexual activity before any rejection occurs. Your warmth and love will be needed to reassure your partner that he or she is still very much desired by you.

Caution
Watch out for the vicious cycle that can wreck sexual pleasure when chronic arthritic pain reduces sexual interest and the ensuing loss of interest leads to depression. The depression itself can make the pain worse. The anticipation and fear of pain can be more devastating to sexual relations than the illness.

Tip
Your partner can try pain-relieving techniques before starting sexual relations: a warm bath or shower, compresses to affected joints. With physician's approval, pain medication may be taken before engaging in sexual activity.

Interestingly, in some situations sexual intercourse seems to relieve arthritic pain and depression. In fact, after orgasm many arthritics feel pain relief for up to thirty minutes. A physician at the Human Sexuality Teaching Program at New York Hospital-Cornell Medical Center, in New York, suggests, "Sexual activity, especially orgasms, stimulates the pleasure zone of the brain; probably endorphins are released giving an analgesic effect."

Mobility problems may be eased by a steady, medically approved program of exercise.

Diabetes Mellitus

Common concerns
Your partner may worry that the diabetes will affect his or her sexual functioning. This is a valid cause for worry because diabetes in some cases does have certain consequences that can cause difficulties. A significant number of diabetic men experience erectile, ejaculatory, and/or impotence problems. Some women report difficulty in vaginal lubrication and/or orgasm difficulties.

Caution

Yes, some diabetics encounter sexual difficulties, but a diagnosis of diabetes does not automatically mean trouble. In fact, psychological reactions to anticipated sexual problems can bring on dysfunction.

Tip

Professional guidance may be needed to determine whether or not difficulties are caused by the diabetic's condition. Counseling can prove invaluable to help bring your partner to his or her optimum level of sexual functioning. In appropriate cases where counseling alone does not help impotency problems, penile implants may be an alternative to consider.

Disfiguring Facial Surgery

Common fears

The face is the center of our physical expression. It is the number one way we have to show our feelings. Its appearance often plays a major role in attracting others. Obviously, when injury or surgery leave behind facial deformities, your loved one may be traumatized. He or she may feel undesirable or embarrassed. His or her sense of personal identity may be badly shaken. It is a common reaction for such patients to want to withdraw— perhaps from work, social situations, and you. Still, there are some who react in the opposite manner by becoming hypersexual.

Caution

As with any type of disfiguring surgery, reactions vary. Your partner may be in emotional trouble if he or she experiences persistent depression, withdrawal, thoughts of suicide, sexual disturbances, and/or avoids returning to work. If you are having trouble coping with your loved one's changed appearance both of you may benefit by asking for help from a mental health professional.

Hysterectomy

Common concerns

For many women hysterectomy is emotionally unsettling. For some it can be devastating. They see the uterus not only as a child-bearing organ, but also as a sexual organ—the core of their femininity, sexual attractiveness, and womanly strength. After hysterectomy your partner may feel that her femininity has been compromised, that she is no longer a "whole woman." At such times she may need much reassurance from you. She needs to know that she is very much desired and loved, that none of her femininity has been lost.

Although surgery may affect your partner emotionally, it should have no effect on the physical side of sexual functioning.

Caution

Depression and other emotional difficulties that appear after this surgery are reasons for concern. Sexual disturbances are most often due to irrational fears and psychological effects of surgery in the genital area.

Tip

Your loved one may benefit from a support group where she can discuss her feelings with other women who have had similar types of surgery. If cancer was found during surgery she may have additional fears. Get in touch with your local cancer society or social worker to locate support groups in your community.

Open Heart Surgery

Common concerns

Your partner may wonder: Will sex harm the chest or the breast bone? Will sex be too fatiguing? Will sex be good or bad for the heart? These are natural fears, but rarely things to worry about. A physician can tell you when to resume the pattern of sexual behavior enjoyed before surgery.

Caution
Certain sexual positions may be uncomfortable for your loved one, especially if the chest area is still sensitive. Experiment to find positions that are the most comfortable and put least strain on the body.

Pregnancy should be postponed until your loved one has recovered completely from surgery. Most physicians suggest waiting at least a year to avoid the intense physical stress of pregnancy. Furthermore, some contraceptives are not advisable for heart patients. Check with your medical advisor.

Tip
You and your partner may feel some tension and uneasiness about sex after open-heart surgery. You both may benefit if you take more time to hug and caress and get reacquainted with one another gradually.

After Heart Attack

Common concerns
You and your loved one may worry that sex will cause another heart attack. In most cases sexual relations between married couples will not harm the heart. In fact, marital sex takes nearly the same energy as a brisk walk or climbing the stairs. Ask the physician when it will be safe for your partner to resume the sexual activities he or she was accustomed to prior to the heart attack. Know that most people who have been treated successfully for heart attack soon regain the same desire for sex they previously had.

Caution
After a heart attack some individuals may experience fast heart action or symptoms of angina pectoris during sexual intercourse. Most often, these symptoms do not preclude the sex act. If your loved one has these symptoms ask the physician what precautions should be taken. Also, research suggests that extramarital sex

can place a greater strain on the heart than sex with one's spouse. In fact, extramarital sex can produce increased elevated heart rate and blood pressure.

Tip

It may be wise to reduce the physical exertion of sexual activity by trying different positions that are easier for your partner. For example, the side to side position is often ideal. Or when the man has had the heart attack, try the female-on-top.

Mastectomy

Common concerns

Your loved one may be experiencing a constellation of feelings: Was all the cancer removed? Is my life in danger? How will my husband react? How will I explain myself to a new lover? Will my figure look different in clothes? She may mourn the loss of her breast. She may feel like damaged goods or mutilated. Some women, fearing rejection by their partners, withdraw from relationships, rejecting themselves before anyone else does.

Does a mastectomy hamper a woman's sexual functioning? Definitely not. Orgasm does not change. Lubrication of the vagina does not cease. And sexual drive is not reduced. It is an old wives' tale that mastectomy causes physical dysfunction.

However, for many women loss of a breast can cause emotional problems—and that can interfere with a woman's sexual life. A British study in 1980 found that 50% of the mastectomy patients surveyed had sexual difficulties. This figure shot up to 70% when the women surveyed had undergone both mastectomy and chemotherapy.

Caution

Mastectomy can produce a great many negative feelings in women who undergo this surgery—and this can affect their sexual functioning. Yet many physicians are so concerned with caring for their patients' physical health that they forget about their mental health. Time does not necessarily heal the emotional repercussions of this surgery. Therefore, any woman who has persistent emotional problems (depression, anxiety, loss of sexual interest, thoughts of suicide, etc.) should consider seeking professional help.

Some men may be fearful about resuming sexual relations with their lovers because they fear they will hurt them. This is a dangerous situation. It can underscore the woman's own anxieties about injury and self-image. If a man does not explain his fears to his lover, she may read them as a rejection, not concern. Communication between partners about each other's fears and thoughts can help a lot to ease sexual tensions.

Tip
One of the best ways for a woman to heal her emotional wounds is to join a support group made up of others who have had mastectomies. Here, women share feelings and experiences. They ventilate and release pent-up emotions. They learn coping skills. To find the one nearest you contact your local cancer society, YWCA, self-help hotline or the National Self-Help Clearinghouse. Note: Do not confuse support groups with the Reach-to-Recovery Program sponsored by the American Cancer Society. This program, generally speaking, helps women who are *in* the hospital. Support groups are meant for after-care.

Ostomy Surgery

Common concerns
This surgery changes the appearance of the lower gastrointestinal tract or the urinary tract by creating an artificial opening (called the stoma) on the abdomen and diverting the usual flow of intestinal contents or urine.

Yes, there is a change in body appearance after this type of surgery. But consider that the operation brings with it many positive benefits. No longer chronically ill, your loved one may have a renewed desire for the closeness of a sexual relationship. True, the stoma may require some adjustment, but its existence may allow your loved one new freedom and energy for sexual pleasuring.

At the same time, your partner may question his or her sexual attractiveness after surgery because of the surgical scar and stoma. He or she may worry that you will be repelled. Your partner may be very concerned about the possibility of unpleasant stomal odors, the appliance, or the appearance of the stoma itself.

Your loved one may also be afraid that the ostomy surgery will affect sexual functioning. Clearly, much of the discussion your partner has had with medical professionals prior to the procedure was about stoma care, diet considerations—and probably little about sexuality. Therefore, it's not unlikely that he or she may have concocted a set of uninformed conclusions.

Caution

There are several different ostomies: ileostomy, colostomy, and ileal conduit (sometimes called urostomy, see Chapter 7). A significant number of post-surgical sexual problems are emotionally rather than physically induced. It is essential that your partner ask the physician how, if at all, the ostomy surgery will affect sexual functioning. If the physician is not forthcoming with such information, consult another or get help at a human sexuality clinic of the type mentioned earlier in this chapter.

Patients who have had extensive surgery that has resulted in nerve damage because of removal of cancerous tissue may encounter physical sexual problems. For men, these difficulties may include erectile and ejaculatory trouble. For women, effects may include painful intercourse, diminished pelvic sensations, and orgasm problems.

As the patient's sexual partner it is important that you be exposed to the meaning of the surgery, the stoma, and the appliance from the beginning. Talk to the physician so that you know what to expect and how best to support your loved one.

Your partner should wait a sufficient amount of time to regain strength before resuming sexual intercourse. However, cuddling and stroking need not be stopped and can be wonderful medicine. Consult the physician about the appropriate time to resume intercourse. Clearly, a person who begins sexual intercourse too soon risks a disappointing experience that may only undermine his or her confidence and self-esteem.

Remember, too, that certain medications for ostomates can affect sexual functioning. Turn to the medical professional for advice.

Tip

Men who are impotent after an ostomy may want to consider having a test to determine if the reason for their problem is emotionally or physically induced. The test checks nocturnal penile tumescence patterns. Simply stated, the procedure is done in a laboratory setting. The erectile movements of the penis are monitored while the man sleeps. Absence of erections during sleep may strongly suggest that the cause of impotence is physical. Only highly trained and experienced professionals can decide conclusively.

When impotence has a permanent physical cause the male ostomate may want to consider penile implants to restore erection.

Women in their childbearing years should know that ostomy does not, generally, interfere with the ability to become pregnant or deliver a healthy baby. In addition, if oral contraceptives are the contraceptives of choice the female ostomate should check with the physician to be sure that this is an effective method of birth control. The reason: Because of the ostomate's surgery the oral contraceptive may not be properly absorbed into the body for optimal effectiveness.

Consider different positions during sex if you are concerned about contact with the stoma during sexual activity. Suggestions include rear entry, female-on-top, side-to-side with the pouch (appliance) closest to the bed.

Many ostomates are afraid that stomal odors and pouch noises

will offend their sex partners. For ileostomates and colostomates common odor-producing foods to beware of include beans, onions, asparagus, some medications, eggs, fish, cheese, and cabbage. Some gas-causing foods are beans, onions, cabbage, beer. People who have had an ileal conduit (urostomy) can usually have a regular diet with few if any restrictions. Know that cranberry juice can help fight urinary odors.

To muffle pouch sounds, encase the bag in a commercially available or self-made covering. Avoid gas-causing foods.

Empty collection pouch before sex play. Your loved one may want to consider a smaller disposable pouch or a new clean one to use only during sexual activity. Concerned ostomates may leave a scented perfumed cotton ball or scented bathroom tissue (Charmin, White Cloud, etc.) inside pouch to reduce noise and odors.

Bismuth subsalicylate or bismuth subgallate with meals is often helpful in controlling unattractive pouch smells. Check with physician.

Your partner may want to secure the pouch to his or her abdomen with surgical tape before strenuous sexual activity to decrease the risk of the bag coming loose or pulling off.

Prostate Surgery

Common concerns
Many men believe that after prostate surgery they will no longer be able to have sex. Such anxiety usually does more damage to sex lives than the surgery itself. Fortunately, for most men sexual desire, performance and pleasure return within several months after surgery. In fact, if your loved one had a severely enlarged prostate, his general health may be vastly improved after surgery, and this may improve his sex life.

Caution
Ask the physician exactly how the surgery will affect your partner's sexual functioning. Such knowledge is imperative so

that your partner can make an informed choice about surgery. In most cases post-operative impotence is emotionally induced. However, some men will experience erectile problems after prostate surgery. This is more likely after open prostate surgery (when an incision is made in the abdomen) than with TUR (transurethral resection: surgery is done through the urethra). A radical prostatectomy almost always causes impotence. This extensive surgery is prescribed to remove cancerous tissue. So the benefits of a radical procedure should be weighed against the impotence that may result.

One more thing: Some men may notice a change after surgery even when sex seems just fine. What's the change? Their orgasm may feel as it did before surgery, but now the ejaculation flows backwards into the bladder creating a "dry" climax. Sperm is still produced in the testicles, but this irregular ejaculation may cause problems when the man wants to father a child. Your medical professional will have to help you with this problem.

Stroke

Common concerns

Your patient may be afraid that sexual activity will produce stress so severe that it will lead to another stroke and possibly death. This is a natural concern, but it is groundless.

In addition, the stroke may have caused some physical or emotional changes in your patient that could affect his or her sex life. These include loss of sensation, paralysis, personality changes, speech and visual impairments, and depression. Know that most physical and emotional difficulties following a stroke can be overcome with professional counseling and rehabilitation.

Caution

For many stroke patients depression is a major sexual saboteur. The person who feels depressed after a stroke may be upset that he or she is not as active or as strong as before. He or she may mourn the loss of function that may have occurred. Let your

loved one know that he or she means as much to you as ever. Encourage your partner to express his or her feelings. This can help ease fear and loneliness.

It is not unusual for the male lover of a woman who has had a stroke to experience impotence. This can happen when the man is afraid that he will hurt his lover, that sex will cause another stroke, or that sexual relations are improper at this time. In most instances, if the couple's sex life was satisfactory before illness, this problem will gradually fade. If it persists, however, professional help may be necessary.

Tip

The need for physical closeness—touching, caressing, embracing, talking—is especially important for the stroke patient. It's doubly important when the stroke victim's own communication abilities—such as speech and sight—have been impaired. Intimacy can reassure the individual that he or she is still cared for and loved.

The degree of disability depends on the severity of the stroke. If your loved one has mobility problems, a trapeze over the bed or a handle on the headboard can make movement easier for him or her during sex play.

What can you do when weakness or paralysis of the body makes the missionary position difficult for the man who has had a stroke? Try the male supine position.

It is beneficial to touch your partner's stroke-involved side. Although there may be a sensation loss, your loved one may feel pressure. Just as important, he or she will see that you are recognizing and accepting the stroke-involved side.

Spinal Injuries

Common concerns

A partner with spinal cord injury may worry that his or her lack of mobility and/or loss of sensation will make sex exceed-

ingly difficult or even impossible. Without question, professional counseling and support can enable such an individual to regain confidence.

Caution

Quadraplegic individuals whose spinal cord injury is at or above the fifth thoracic level are at risk for a potentially dangerous condition called *autonomic hyperreflexia*. It can lead to severe elevations in blood pressure, which if untreated can result in convulsions, even death. Any physical stimulation, such as constipation, catheterization, bladder distention, and stimulation of the genitals, can bring on this condition. If your loved one is a quadraplegic, he or she may have experienced such an attack at least once and know how to recognize its signs: excessive sweating, slowing of heart, shivering and goose bumps, flushing of skin, dilation of pupils with accompanying irritation from bright lights, blurred vision, and severe pounding headache.

The condition is treated by finding the source of the irritation and removing it. Clearly, when a specific type of activity is the cause (direct stimulation of the head of the penis or clitoris, etc.) it should be stopped. A person with a spinal cord injury should communicate this possibility to his or her partner. In some cases medication is prescribed to reduce the frequency and severity of attacks.

Tip

Professional counseling can be invaluable when it comes to helping the person who has a spinal cord injury recover his or her sexual potential. There are many publications on this subject, See the earlier section of this chapter for addresses. In addition, there is a helpful book called *The Sensuous Wheeler*, by Barry Rabin, Ph.D. Write for it to Multimedia Bookstore, 1525 Franklin St., San Francisco, Calif. 99409.

Impotence: Scientific Breakthroughs

If your partner is experiencing erectile and/or ejaculatory difficulties that are interfering with sexual performance and pleasure there are care alternatives he may want to consider.

First, it is important that the reason for impotence be determined. Is it emotionally or physically induced? There are times when the physician or urologist will be able to pinpoint the cause; but when this is not possible, or when their diagnosis is not satisfactory to you or your loved one, contact a human sexuality clinic affiliated with a major hospital. Or consult a certified sex therapist, as discussed earlier in this chapter. These resources can direct you to the professionals who can perform the type of examinations and tests needed to determine the cause of the problem. Once the cause is discovered, proper medical treatment and/or therapy can be provided.

There are a variety of diagnostic tests that can be given to better understand your partner's potential. One of the most common is the nocturnal penile tumescence test. As discussed earlier, this test records a man's erectile activity while he sleeps. Since the average male experiences erections during sleep, an absence of such activity as recorded in the NPT test suggests a physical reason for impotence. Other tests may be made to determine if there is a circulatory problem causing difficulties. Vascular surgery is sometimes performed to correct circulatory problems in appropriate individuals. When the cause of impotence is clearly a circulatory one, such a procedure may be indicated, but naturally it should be performed by a highly qualified and experienced surgeon.

Another procedure to be considered when impotence is caused by physical problems is the penile prosthesis. Simply stated, this device is surgically implanted in the penis to create an artificial erection.

There are several types of prostheses. For example, one type involves the insertion of semirigid silicone rods into the penis that result in a permanent erection. Another type is an inflatable model. Here, when an erection is desired the man manipulates a pumping mechanism that has been implanted in the scrotal pouch.

Penile prostheses can restore the ability to have sexual intercourse. However, this surgery should be considered only for patients whose impotence has proved to be physically caused or when sex therapy fails. Although there has been much success with these surgical procedures, know that they result in a somewhat shorter, thinner, and more flexible penis.

To answer your questions about impotence, sexuality, and sexual problems, and to receive referrals to experienced and competent professionals contact The National Sex Forum, 1523 Franklin St., San Francisco, Calif. 94109. Or you may call their Sexual Health Care Clinic for immediate advice and referrals at (415) 928-1208. Next door to the National Sex Forum is the Multimedia Bookstore, which distributes a wide range of books on human sexuality. For their publication list, write to the Multimedia Bookstore, 1525 Franklin St., San Francisco, Calif. 94109.

On the East Coast you can call the Community Sex Information hotline in New York City. This service can provide immediate advice and referrals. Call Monday through Thursday, 6:00 P.M. to 8:00 P.M. at (212) 677-3320.

Two books to consider are *Impotence: Physiological, Psychological and Surgical Diagnosis and Treatment*, by Gorm Wagner and Richard Green, New York: Plenum Press, 1982 (this book is geared toward medical professionals with the latest information on the subject) and *Lifelong Sexual Vision: How to Avoid and Overcome Impotence*, by Marvin and Sally Brooks, New York: Doubleday, 1981 (this book is directed toward medical consumers).

Gay individuals may want to contact the National Gay Task Force in New York City. This organization has extensive listing of medical programs and support groups sympathetic to the concerns of gay men and women. Call (212) 741-5800.

A Word About Reproductive Health Care
and Family Planning

Many disabilities do not interfere with a woman's ability to conceive or a man's ability to father a child. Therefore, the issue of family planning remains an important one.

Equally as important is the subject of reproductive health care. For example, women should have regular Pap smears and breast and gynecological examinations. Men require regular urological and prostate examinations.

Discuss these issues with the physician. To get more information and/or to locate your local Planned Parenthood Center write to The Reproductive Health Care and Disability Program c/o Planned Parenthood of New York City, Margaret Sanger Center, 380 Second Ave., New York, N.Y. 10010, att: Coordinator.

10

Emergency Medical Care: Life-Saving Steps for Your Patient

Patients have suffered and some have died needlessly because their care givers didn't know how to provide proper emergency treatment. If the thought of a health crisis sends waves of fright up your spine, let me suggest that the best way to allay your fears, and possibly save your loved one's life, is to be prepared.

Would you know what to do if your patient suddenly had breathing difficulties, started to bleed profusely, or fell unconscious? Would you know who to call for help? Or, if necessary, how to transport your patient to the hospital emergency room?

You must have an emergency plan for your patient—one worked out ahead of time with a medical professional so that a health crisis does not turn into unnecessary anguish or tragedy. Here's the five-step plan that can get you started.

Five Steps for Ever-ready Emergency Care

1. Know the medical emergencies that can arise from your patient's condition. Ask the physician to list them for you.

2. Ask the physician what to do in the event that an anticipated emergency occurs.

3. Know how to perform the life-saving techniques that may

227

be needed. For example, if your patient has swallowing difficulties you should know the anti-choking technique called the
Heimlich Maneuver. If the patient is at risk for heart attack, know
how to administer the artificial respiration and circulation technique called Cardio-Pulmonary Resuscitation. Learn how to perform these life-saving procedures from medical professionals such
as the physician or nurse or take the special training courses
offered in your community.

4. Have a complete list of emergency numbers taped by your
telephone. They should include: physician (numbers that allow
access to him/her twenty-four hours a day); hospital emergency
room; ambulance service; paramedic or cardiac service (if one
exists in your area); poison control; pharmacy; nurse and/or nursing service; local police department; local fire department; dentist,
nearby neighbor who can help; nearest relative to call, if necessary.

5. Prepare a medical record that can be carried with the patient
to the emergency room. This can provide the emergency medical
staff with invaluable information about your patient's condition
and medical history. Important information to include: patient's
name, address, current medical problems, medication taken regularly, dangerous allergies, last immunization dates (tetanus tox-
oid, diphtheria, small pox, measles, polio, typhoid, etc.), and a
reduced copy of the electrocardiogram (EKG), especially for patients with a history of heart problems. Also, get your patient a
Medic Alert Emblem. This necklace or bracelet is engraved with
a statement of the patient's condition and a phone number to be
called for additional information. The Medic Alert Emblem can
be a life-saver when the patient cannot speak because of unconsciousness, shock, delirium, hysteria, loss of articulation, or other
debilitating conditions. For additional information write Medic
Alert Foundation International, P.O. Box 1009, Turlock, Calif.
95380.

What Is an Emergency?

Some care givers have trouble recognizing life-threatening situations. To identify these moments more easily refer to the following list and consult the physician.

Life-threateners:
• breathing difficulties (congestive heart failure, pulmonary edema, asthma, etc.)
• shock
• heart-attack symptoms (chest pains, etc.)
• unconsciousness
• possible poisonings
• severe allergic reactions
• diabetic shock or coma
• choking
• stroke
• spinal injuries
• dehydration
• uncontrollable bleeding
• internal bleeding
• major burns
• others indicated by the physician that relate to your patient's condition

To Call the Ambulance or Not To?

This isn't always an easy question to answer for two goo reasons. First, you may wonder whether or not your patient condition is serious enough to warrant an ambulance. Second, you are unsure of the quality of services available, you may l reluctant to hand over your patient's care to strangers. These ar natural concerns that are easily alleviated with a bit of knowledge.

Ambulances are best for true emergencies because they are fitted with special equipment. They can, generally speaking, weave through traffic quickly. Their staffs have been specially trained to provide care—and not to panic.

On the other hand, in some areas ambulance service is noto-
riously slow, of poor quality, or both. Check with the physician
or nurse to find out which ambulance services they recommend
for your patient.

It's possible that your patient's best bet is a car or taxi ride
instead of an ambulance to an emergency care facility. If you are
torn between calling an ambulance or driving the patient to the
hospital in a car or taxi note the following guidelines.

Call an ambulance if:
• your patient is unconscious
• you think your patient has had a stroke
• your patient is having severe breathing difficulties
• your patient has a broken back or neck
• you are too panicked to drive safely or cope
• your patient is bleeding severely (internally or externally)
• your patient may have had a heart attack. Here an ambulance
may be equipped to handle this emergency, but time is of the
essence. If you suspect the ambulance will take too long, use an
alternative method.

What to Tell the Ambulance Dispatcher

In the words of one paramedic, "Want to know the most common mistake care givers make when they call for an ambulance?
They call the service, describe their patient's problem, but hang
up before giving the dispatcher their address."

Panic can make us very absent-minded—and that's a luxury
few can afford during a health emergency. So to prevent foolish
mistakes that can jeopardize your patient's life, be sure you give
the ambulance dispatcher the following information.
• Give your patient's name and address.
• Give the address of the emergency—with landmarks to help
the driver find it as fast as possible.
• Describe what's wrong with the patient so that the ambulance
can be better prepared upon arrival.

• After you call the ambulance, call the physician. He can give you additional care instructions while you are waiting for help.

• It may help to have someone available to flag down the ambulance, if possible.

Ambulances: What Kinds Are There?

You'll have an easier time picking the best ambulance service for your patient if you know what's available. Here's a rundown of the most common types.

• Hospital ambulances are dispatched from specific hospitals to pick up patients and to bring them back to the hospital. If you opt for this service, be sure that you have the phone number handy. There is usually a fee.

• City ambulances are dispatched by city hospitals to pick up patients and bring them back to the nearest city, public, or hospital. To call one, use the three-digit emergency number in your city. For many cities it is 911. Know yours. (Check with your local operator.) In most places a call to the local fire department or police will bring an ambulance. City ambulances are provided as a service to the public so you usually don't have to pay.

• Private services take you to the hospital of your choice. Quality varies, so ask your physician for a referral to a reputable service. Private ambulances are often expensive and require on-the-spot payment. However, your patient's health insurance may cover costs. Check the policy. (Know that these services do not always provide paramedical care.)

Home-Care Patients Who Live Alone: Emergency Alternatives

Perhaps you cannot be with your patient all day long or maybe you know a sick person who lives alone. What can these people do if they suddenly, because of a health crisis, have difficulty communicating on the phone to get help?

In some parts of the country the telephone company offers "Speed Calling." With it your patient can reach emergency or frequently called numbers faster—even long distance numbers— by *dialing only one or two digits*. Contact your local telephone business office for more information.

Also, there are push-button alarm systems that can be installed in your patient's home to dispatch immediate medical ambulance assistance. These services supply ambulances twenty-four hours a day, every day. Naturally, you'll want to be sure that the service provided is excellent and offers fast transport to the best facility. For more information, check the Yellow Pages under "Alarms," or "Medical Alarms," ask the physician, or write Emergency Medical Alert System, 1678 East 31st St., Brooklyn, N.Y. 11234.

Which Emergency Room Is Best?

You don't want to rely on guesswork at the last minute to decide where to take your patient in an emergency. Again, ask the physician for a recommendation. In certain circumstances, it's wise to choose a hospital where the physician has privileges. In this way, if your patient needs to be admitted for hospital care, the next step is a simple move upstairs to the right floor.

Ideally, you will want to locate the nearest emergency room with twenty-four-hour service and a physician on duty. If feasible, try for a large teaching hospital as they often have top-notch emergency facilities.

What You Can Expect in the Emergency Room

The medical professional on duty will decide who needs medical care first. Generally, patients are treated in the order they arrive. However, seriously ill or injured patients are given top priority.

Stay calm if you have accompanied your loved one to the emergency room. You may be needed to clearly and quickly explain the reason for your patient's visit.

What about emergency room fees? In most cases they include a basic charge for the treatment room and physician, and additional charges for tests, X rays, medication, and special treatments. These charges are often covered by health insurance policies.

Your Emergency Care Support Guide

The drawback of many emergency-care guides and first-aid books is that they tend to give their readers a false sense of security. Chances are, a few well-written paragraphs and some deftly drawn diagrams will not be enough to get you through a full-blown medical emergency. That's why you should consider getting instruction directly from medical professionals.

Let me offer you an example: me. For the longest time I believed that I could perform CPR—a life-saving technique that can help restore breathing and blood circulation—by referring to a book. When a CPR demonstration was offered at the company where I worked I realized that the procedure was a bit more difficult than I had thought. So I took a course in CPR at a local hospital. Without question, professional instruction and supervision enabled me to learn and perform the maneuver with confidence and accuracy. My advice: Get professional instruction to perform the techniques that may be needed to save your loved one's life. I believe that every home-care giver should learn CPR and the Heimlich Maneuver (an aid for choking victims). Contact the physician to help you find low-cost or free instruction in your community. Other sources of advice include nurses, local Red Cross chapters, fire departments, or local hospitals.

Miniguide to Emergency Care

The miniguide that follows should provide you with emergency support during a variety of home-care emergencies. It is not a substitute for professional instruction. Use it as a reference and consult the physician or nurse for additional guidance.

Bleeding

External bleeding

Possible causes of abnormal external bleeding are recent surgery, injury, and reopening of a wound.

• If your patient is bleeding from a wound dressing, apply pressure to the site. If bleeding has restarted, call physician immediately for advice. Describe the amount of bleeding and other associated signs such as fever, pain, and odor from the wound site.

• If your patient bleeds after oral surgery, ask physician ahead of time how much bleeding to expect. A small amount is usually normal. For example, a cotton change twice a day is often expected for the first two days at home after surgery. If bleeding persists, however, call your physician. Profuse bleeding requires immediate medical attention.

• If your patient bleeds after nasal surgery, ask your physician how much bleeding to expect. Call the doctor if you notice a change or if there is an odor.

• If your patient has a profuse nosebleed, ask him or her to keep the head upright to stop bleeding. Squeeze the nostrils closed so that the patient is breathing through the mouth. Then, wedge gauze pad or cotton between the upper teeth and lip. If profuse bleeding persists, take the patient to a hospital emergency room.

• If your patient is bleeding profusely from an external wound, apply direct pressure to the site with gauze, clean cotton, or cloth. If bleeding is severe, put the patient's feet up higher than the site of injury to help blood get to the heart. Call the physician and give this information: location of bleeding, amount of blood, other signs, blood pressure, what precipitated bleeding. If you have an oxygen supply at home, give the patient oxygen and keep him or her warm. Don't give anything to drink, or eat as this can cause choking if the patient becomes unconscious.

Internal bleeding

Possible causes of internal bleeding are recent surgery, injury, ulcers, anticoagulant therapy, chemotherapy, and hemophilia.

Internal bleeding usually means bleeding into the abdominal or pelvic area, chest, or other organ.

• If you suspect internal bleeding, watch for telltale signs: paleness, cold, clammy skin, blood-pressure drop, rapid pulse, restlesness, faintness, shallow irregular breathing, anxiety. In addition, there may be pain at the site, patient may be vomiting blood, have black, tarry stool, blood in stool, or urine. Internal bleeding is serious and requires immediate medical intervention. The danger is that the patient can go into life-threatening shock.

• If your patient has vaginal bleeding, do not confuse it with normal menstrual bleeding. Spotting should be brought to the physician's attention. This, however, is rarely an emergency. But if the patient is pregnant and has a sudden onset of vaginal bleeding, this is an emergency. Call the physician and get your patient to a hospital emergency room. In cases of cancer or recent gynecologic surgery, call the physician at once or take your patient to the hospital emergency room. If your patient has pain associated with vaginal bleeding, call the physician immediately for advice.

• If your patient has rectal bleeding, watch for bright red blood mixed with stool, which may mean hemorrhoids. Note black, tarry stool. This may mean that internal bleeding is higher up. Internal bleeding is a serious sign and requires prompt medical evaluation. Call for professional advice if you have questions.

Cardio-Pulmonary Resuscitation

Use when:
• patient has stopped breathing
• patient may be in cardiac arrest. The signs of cardiac arrest are absence of pulse in the carotid arteries on both sides of the neck, unconsciousness, no breathing, and/or a deathlike look.

Tips
Consider purchasing a CPR kit or improvise one yourself. A commercial kit will contain plastic airways (adult and child-sized)

Figure 9. Cardiopulmonary Resuscitation

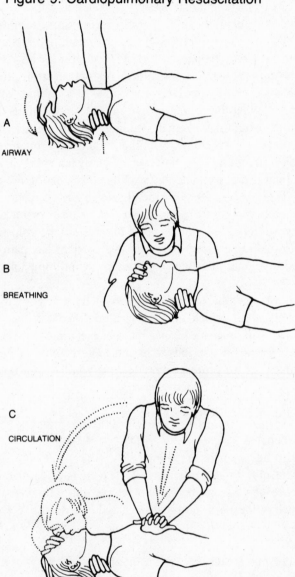

A

AIRWAY

B

BREATHING

C

CIRCULATION

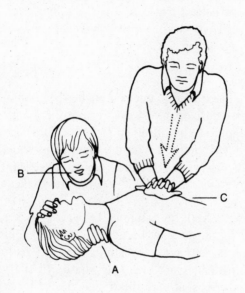

CPR TECHNIQUE*

one rescuer
15 compressions
  (80 per minute)
2 quick breaths
depress sternum
  1½ to 2 inches

two rescuers
5 compressions
  (60 per minute)
1 breath

*Continue procedure without stopping until advanced life support is available, or until respiration and pulse return.

which are inserted into the patient's mouth. These airways protect you from contamination by keeping the patient's tongue down and providing unobstructed air flow. They appeal to some care givers because they eliminate the need for direct mouth-to-mouth contact between patient and care giver. . . . Know that there are special considerations when performing CPR on infants and children. Consult physician for advice.

What to do
1. Airway. Place your patient on his/her back on a hard surface. If unconscious, open airway. Perform neck tilt (see illustration: A in Figure 9) by lifting up patient's neck with one hand and pushing down forehead with the other. This should be sufficient to open airway. If you see a foreign body fish it out with your fingers. Remove foreign matter from mouth, including dentures.

2. Breathing. Check for breathing by watching chest rise and fall, listening for air passing through the nose or mouth, feeling for air from nose or mouth. Breathing may be shallow, so be alert. If your patient is not breathing, start artificial respiration by pinching nostrils shut with the fingers of one hand and blow into mouth (see illustration: B). Be sure that the air you are blowing does not leak out from around the patient's mouth or through the nose. For first artificial respirations, attempt four fast, full breaths into the patient. Check chest for expansion. (For infants and children, cover both nose and mouth with your mouth and use smaller, less forceful breaths to get air into lungs. Inflate once every three seconds.)

3. Circulation. Check carotid pulse (large arteries at either side of neck). To find: Go to the Adam's apple, feel on either side of it one side at a time for pulse. If pulse is nonexistent, start artificial circulation (see illustration: C). Two very fast lung inflations are given after each fifteen chest compressions. For one rescuer: You must perform both breathing *and* circulation. For two rescuers: One person can perform external cardiac massage while the other does respiration (see illustration).

Choking

Serious consequences can result when food is sucked into the windpipe instead of being swallowed, or any object becomes accidentally lodged in it.

What to do

If the person can talk, it is best to let him or her cough up the object without interference. If the person cannot talk, communicate, or breathe, start Heimlich Maneuver as detailed below (see Figure 10: A).

The standing victim:

1. Stand behind the person and clasp your arms around the waist.
2. Allow upper body to hang forward.
3. Grab your fist with your other hand and place the thumb side of your fist against the victim's abdomen, slightly above the navel and below the rib cage.
4. Press your fist sharply into the abdomen using a fast, upward thrust. Do these movements several times if necessary.

The lying down victim:

1. If the person is lying on his or her back, face and kneel astride thighs, turning head to side to prevent aspiration of foreign objects into lungs. With one hand on top of the other, place the heel of your bottom hand on the abdomen slightly above the navel and below the rib cage (see illustration: B).
2. Press forcefully into the abdomen with a quick upward thrust toward head.

When the victim is a small child:

Try to remove food or foreign object from your child's airway by turning the little one upside down over one arm and giving blows to the back between the shoulder blades (see illustration: C). Moderate force of blows.

Figure 10. The Heimlich Maneuver for Choking

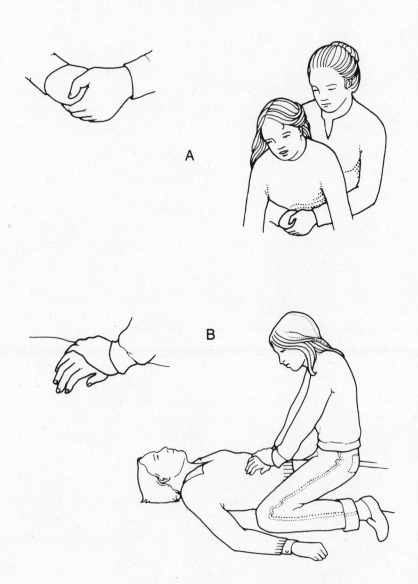

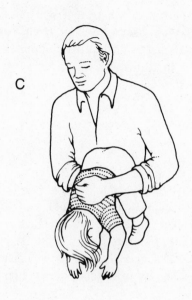

C

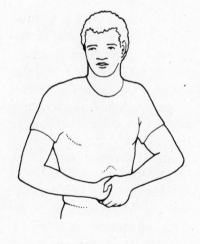

D

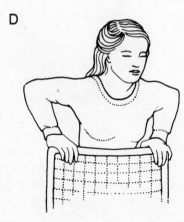

When you are alone:

You want to do anything that will push forceably into your abdomen. Try the back of a chair, your own fist, or some other object at abdomen level (see illustration: D).

The object in all instances is to force the diaphragm upwards, pressing air into the lungs and ejecting the object from the windpipe.

Diabetic Emergencies

Insulin or hypoglycemic reaction (too little sugar in the blood) may occur because the patient took too much insulin, didn't eat at all, didn't eat enough, or had too much exercise. It may happen suddenly, but often there are warning signs. The patient breaks out in a sweat, feels shaky, has headache, feels out of sorts, confused or hungry; no fruity odor on breath.

What to do

Give your patient skim milk as it produces a gradual and sustained correction of blood without overshooting the mark. It has also been traditional to use orange juice, sugar, or hard candy, but many authorities feel that milk is a better choice if warning signs are picked up early. Then consult a physician. Do not give any foods or liquids to an unconscious patient. If the patient is unconscious get immediate medical help by calling an ambulance or taking him or her to an emergency room.

Diabetic coma may result when there is too much sugar in the blood and ketones—breakdown products in the metabolism of fat—that tend to accumulate in the insulin-dependent diabetic. It may occur because your patient didn't take enough of the prescribed medication, overate, or has an infection or illness. It happens gradually. Early warning signs are excessive urination and extreme thirst. If treatment is not given quickly these signs will appear: nausea, vomiting, deep rapid breathing, dry tongue, fruity breath, dry and flushed skin. Coma will occur if treatment is not administered at once.

What to do
Get immediate medical help. If this is not possible, give insulin by injection. Call doctor for appropriate amount. If neither insulin nor medical help are on hand, treat your patient as if he/she is in shock. Give large amounts of liquids by mouth, but do not give sugar, carbohydrates, or fats in any form. Do not give any food or liquid to an unconscious person. Call ambulance or get patient to emergency room at once.

Fainting

Your patient may lose consciousness from having seen or heard unpleasant things, or from remaining too long in an upright position. There may be an underlying medical condition, such as heart disease; low blood sugar or low blood pressure can also cause fainting.

What to do
You can prevent loss of consciousness when someone feels faint by laying him or her flat with the head lower than the legs. If the person can't be laid down, assist to a head-between-the-knees position until feelings of faintness pass. Call physician to determine the cause of the episode. Ammonia salts may be used to revive a person who has fainted; purchase at drugstore.

Heart Attack

Heart attack is caused by impaired profusion of the cardiac muscle due to narrowing or spasms of the blood vessels. Some precipitating factors include pulmonary embolism, thyroid disease, emotional distress, and overexertion.

The heart-attack victim may experience sensations of uncomfortable pressure, squeezing, and fullness or pain in the center of the chest behind the breastbone that can spread to the left shoulder, neck, or arm and last for fifteen minutes or more. Other signs include clammy skin, sweating, breathing difficulties, feelings of weakness, nausea, or vomiting. These are classic signs of heart attack, but about 30% of heart-attack victims do not have the classic symptoms.

What to do

Too many heart-attack deaths occur needlessly because victims do not get medical help in time. They may hesitate or worry: *"What if I'm wrong?"* Get medical advice or help quickly. Delay costs lives.

Ask the victim to stop all activity, sit down or lie still, and loosen clothes. If pain lasts longer than fifteen minutes, call a physician or emergency rescue service, or get the victim to the hospital.

If cardiac arrest occurs (no breathing, no pulse) start CPR at once.

If your patient has angina and you suspect heart attack, you should know that angina rarely causes loss of consciousness. Your loved one may clutch his or her chest and have difficulty breathing.

Many patients can feel the difference between the two. Be alert to changes in the pattern of pain, frequency, inducing factors, or increased intensity of pain. These signs are called "unstable angina" and often precede a heart attack. They require prompt medical intervention to prevent a heart attack.

If your patient has a history of angina and nitroglycerine is handy, administer it at once. However, if there are signs of unstable angina as described above and/or your patient is sweating, nauseous, or vomiting, suspect a heart attack and get him or her to the hospital immediately.

Seizures

Convulsions may be due to epilepsy, head injury, medication side effects, high fever, hyperventilation, or infectious illness, especially of the brain. The victim of a seizure may scream or say that he or she sees an "aura," hears something, or senses something is on the verge of happening. He or she usually loses consciousness. The muscles stiffen and then contract, drawing the body into unnatural movement. Breathing may seem to have stopped and the skin may darken.

What to do

1. Stay calm. Watch your patient. A description of what happens during a seizure will help the physician decide the cause of the seizure. For example, is one side affected or all sides? How long did the seizure last?

2. Don't restrain your patient's movements—and don't force any hard objects between the teeth. If possible, place a folded handkerchief or piece of rubber between the teeth to prevent biting of tongue or cheek.

3. Prevent patient from hitting the ground or anything hard. Place pillow or blanket under the head. If necessary, help him or her to a safe place.

4. Turn patient on one side so that he or she does not gag on tongue or vomitus. Loosen tight clothing. Don't give anything to drink. Be sure that he or she can breathe freely.

5. It is rarely necessary to call an ambulance unless a seizure lasts more than ten minutes or is immediately followed by another.

6. Your patient may have some confusion after the seizure. Calmly explain what has happened. Then call the physician for advice. Be sure to notify the physician if this is your patient's first seizure.

Shock

When this condition occurs there is a decrease of the circulating fluids of the blood. This is a life-threatening situation. Unless proper treatment is given, death can result. Therefore, shock needs to be noticed early and handled fast.

Injury, hemorrhage (internal or external), severe burns, infection, allergic reactions, heart attack, stroke, and diabetes are all possibilities for inducing shock. It may also result from drug overdose.

You can't help but notice that something is wrong because your patient will look sick. Usually, there is a group of symptoms: cold, clammy skin, pallor, sunken eyes, rapid, weak, and thready pulse, low blood pressure, mental changes, restlessness, confusion, stupor, coma, reduced urine output, irregular or rapid or shallow respiration. Several or more of these symptoms imply shock.

What to do

Seek immediate medical attention. Alert the emergency room or ambulance staff that you suspect shock so that they are prepared to handle it and administer necessary treatment. In the meantime, while you're waiting for help to arrive, do the following.

1. Keep the patient lying flat and elevate legs about twelve inches by placing a pillow under them.

2. Avoid moving the patient unnecessarily. Transporting the patient must be done properly. The head should be lower than the rest of the body. Keep the patient warm.

3. If an ambulance is unavailable, transport the patient in a car by laying him or her flat on one seat, with legs elevated. Get help to ensure that the patient is moved in a relatively prone position.

Anaphylactic shock is a type of shock that occurs when the body has a hypersensitive reaction to a foreign substance. If the patient's reaction to the offending substance is rapid, fast medical intervention is imperative.

Possible causes of anaphylactic shock are antibiotics (most commonly penicillin, tetracycline, sulfa drugs), allergies, horse serum, hormones, chemicals used in certain diagnostic tests, venom, insect stings, and local anesthetic.

The warning signs are restlessness, swelling of vocal cords, lung congestion, breathing difficulties, severe headache, unconsciousness, severe nausea, vomiting, and diarrhea.

What to do

Get immediate medical help. Until then, ensure that your patient has a clear airway and position the head (see CPR for neck tilt). Patients who are at high risk for anaphylactic shock should have epinephrine nearby. An ANA kit can be purchased at the drugstore. It contains epinephrine, a medication that can bring symptomatic relief to patients in severe allergic states. Ask the medical professional for guidance.

Unconsciousness

Possible causes of unconsciousness are stroke, heart attack, allergic reaction, insulin shock, diabetic coma, bleeding, heat exhaustion, seizure, head injury, suffocation, and accidental or intentional drug overdose.

What to do

If your patient is unconscious, be sure that he or she is still breathing. If not, start artificial respiration at once. Then check the carotid arteries at either side of the neck for the pulse. If there is none, start Cardiopulmonary Resuscitation.

Try to determine the cause of unconsciousness. Call the physician immediately. Even if the patient revives, medical evaluation is essential to determine the reason for loss of consciousness.

Additional sources of information for emergency medical care are listed below.

The American Red Cross
Contact your local office for publications and information about
CPR classes. See phone book for listing.

ACT Foundation
P.O. Box 911
Basking Ridge, N.J. 07920

This is a nonprofit organization that promotes concepts of advanced coronary treatment and sponsors public education and technical assistance programs.

National Association of Emergency Medical Technicians
P.O. Box 334
Newton Highlands, Mass. 02161

This organization provides information to the public about emergency care.

National Registry of Emergency Medical Technicians
P.O. Box 29233
Columbus, Ohio 43229

Here is where you can obtain a list of nationally registered emergency medical technicians if you need to verify a professional's credentials.

11

How to Care for
a Mentally Ill Relative
at Home

Although many of us are unprepared for health catastrophes, we are probably least prepared to care for a loved one who succumbs to mental illness.

Mental illness obliterates normal thoughts and feelings. At times your loved one may seem like a stranger: a chameleon dressed in many colors of mood, action, and, sometimes, bizarre behavior.

When you deal with a mental illness in your family you will encounter feelings of guilt, embarrassment, and loss. You will experience conflicts within the family and you may doubt whether you're doing the right thing.

Although you want to help, you may not get all the assistance and support you need from the professional community. That's where this chapter comes in. Much of the advice and observations on the following pages comes from families and professionals deeply involved in the care of the mentally ill. You will learn that each case is unique and requires its own brand of customized care.

Know that you are not alone in the struggle to help your mentally ill relative. There are millions of Americans engaged in efforts similar to yours. Let this chapter show you how to reach out to find them.

What Is Mental Illness?

The mentally ill individual exhibits an exaggerated behavior that can progress to where it appears peculiar, abnormal, or dangerous. Mental illness can take many forms. Some of the most common will be discussed later in this chapter.

What Types of Mental Illnesses Can Be Managed at Home?

Many cases of mental illness, including depression, schizophrenia, manic depression, and paranoid schizophrenia respond to home treatment. In addition, neurological and physical disorders can cause mental problems in victims of stroke, cancer, Alzheimer's disease, Parkinson's disease, alcoholism, and so on.

When Is Hospital-based Care More Appropriate than Home Care?

The decision to hospitalize a family member for mental illness should be made in collaboration with highly qualified mental health professionals who have assessed your loved one's condition. (There are also legal considerations that vary from state to state.)

Hospital-based care is most appropriate when your relative:
• is a danger to himself/herself and others
• has special needs only a hospital can handle
• is psychotic (out of touch with reality) and unable to recognize that he or she is ill
• refuses medication and treatment to control disturbed symptoms and behavior

• is overwhelming to the care giver and proper home care cannot be provided
  • causes family conflicts that in turn aggravate the illness
  • is suicidal.

When Is Home Care the Right Choice?

Home care should be seriously considered in the following instances.
  • Your ill relative, you, and the mental health professionals assess the condition and decide that competent home care is feasible and can be provided.
  • The ill relative and family get the proper professional support and treatment needed to supervise home care.
  • The home scene does not contain stressful family conflicts or relationships that can aggravate your loved one's condition and cause a relapse.
  • Your loved one is willing to comply with treatment and work cooperatively with the family and mental health professionals.
  • The family is cohesive enough to withstand the disruption, stress, and abnormal behavior that may be displayed by the mentally ill relative.

Who Are the Mental Health Professionals?

Because there are a variety of professionals who provide mental health services, it may be difficult for you to determine who does what. Here's a rundown of professional titles that may clear up some of the confusion.
  • neurologist: This is a medical doctor educated in the treatment of disorders of the nervous system and the brain.
  • psychiatric nurse: This is a registered nurse (R.N.) who has had special training and experience in providing care for the mentally ill.
  • psychiatrist: This is a medical doctor who specializes in the

diagnosis, treatment, and prevention of mental and emotional disturbances. A psychiatrist has a medical degree and four or more years of approved residency training.

• psychoanalyst: This individual is a psychiatrist or psychologist who has had training in the type of psychotherapy developed by Sigmund Freud.

• psychologist: This is a person educated in the science of human behavior and personality. A licensed psychologist has a Ph.D. or its equivalent, two years of supervised experience, and has passed a licensing test. The term "psychologist" and "psychological" can be used to advertise their practice only by licensed psychologists or psychologists who work for federal, state, county, or municipal agencies or schools.

Note: Other professionals who work with the mentally ill include registered nurses and registered therapists and social workers (see Chapter 2). Be sure that you verify the credentials of the professionals(s) caring for your family member. Know the answers to these questions: Where did they go to school? How much post-graduate experience have they had? Are they experienced in caring for people with problems like those of your relative? Because of a lack of consistent laws around the nation, there are lots of unqualified people calling themselves therapists, counselors, group therapists, or psychotherapists. Don't be fooled. Verify qualifications.

How Do You Know Which Mental Health Professional to Turn to?

Chances are your family physician is aware of the most qualified mental health professionals in your community. Ask the physician to refer you to several individuals who may be able to help your relative. Why several? So that you and your patient can "shop around" for the appropriate psychiatrist, psychologist, etc. You see, rapport between the patient and the professional is of prime importance. Furthermore, approach varies among professionals. You will want to locate someone who fits as perfectly as possible with your loved one's mental health needs and personality.

How Will You Know if Your Relative Has Been Diagnosed Properly?

Unfortunately, there are no easy answers. Although enormous strides have been made in treating the mentally ill, there is still much darkness. Professionals can make mistakes. Remember, though, that a sincere, highly qualified professional is likely to prescribe a course of treatment based on reasoning that you, a lay person, may not have considered. If you have reason to question or doubt a professional's approach and/or treatment, ask him or her for an explanation.

What's more, there are certain questions that you can ask yourself to see if your relative is in competent hands.

• Do you see any progress? It may be totally unrealistic, depending on your loved one's condition, to expect mental health to be restored in a short time. In many cases, especially when illness is moderate to severe, progress can be slow. But you should be seeing *some signs* of improvement. Your loved one should be experiencing some relief.

• Does the professional care about your relative and seem committed to his or her growth? You cannot always predict how a professional will conduct him or herself during the period of treatment. However, you should expect the professional to be interested and involved in your loved one's case.

• Does the professional want to help your relative reach his or her own optimum level of mental health? Beware of the professional who approaches your family member as if he or she were a lost cause. This approach is clearly a negative one. And indeed, your loved one may turn into a lost cause if care is administered with an attitude of hopelessness. The overwhelming majority of cases are not lost causes.

• Does your relative feel as if the professional listens to and understands him or her? Certainly, a poor relationship between patient and professional can undermine successful mental-health care. It can also affect the quality of the diagnosis. There is a better chance for a good fit between patient and professional when therapists are screened carefully prior to treatment.

Does Your Relative Insist on a Professional You Don't Approve Of?

Here's another difficult—and not unusual—problem. You may be displeased with the therapist, but you cannot force your opinions on your relative.

The best way to avoid this situation is to carefully screen therapists before treatment. There are, of course, no guarantees, but at least you can glean satisfaction from having tried to secure the best treatment possible.

Another suggestion: Set up an appointment with the professional to express your concerns. In this way, you will make the therapist aware of your misgivings; and sometimes such a conference may reveal that you have misinterpreted the situation and it is not as grim as you had imagined.

How Can You Locate the Right Mental Health Services?

Your community may offer a variety of services for the mentally ill and their families, but finding the service or combination of services you need may be rough.

Seek help from reputable agencies and properly trained and licensed mental health professionals. As I mentioned earlier, you can try referrals from your family physician. Besides that, you may turn to your clergyman, a trusted relative, friend, or social worker.

What Are the Major Problems Facing Home-Care Givers?

Some people who care for mentally ill relatives at home experience feelings of great isolation and helplessness. They believe that their problems are unusual and that no one can understand what they are going through.

Certainly your loved one's condition is special and unique to you, but there are many other care givers and families experiencing problems similar to yours. Perhaps if you know the most common of these problems you won't feel so alone. In the words of a care giver who provided care for her schizophrenic son, "Sometimes care seemed so overwhelming and my son's behavior so upsetting I thought I would lose my mind." The type of stress that you experience will depend on the severity of your loved one's illness and the extent of your coping skills. Here are the stress makers most often cited by the many care givers and mental health professionals I have spoken to.

• embarrassment: Some care givers are troubled by the stigma they associate with mental illness. Other are disconcerted by their loved one's behavior in front of people outside the family.

• responsibility: Here, it's not unusual for some care givers to wonder if they caused their relative's illness. This may be of special concern to parents who fear that their mentally ill child may have inherited the illness.

• twenty-four-hour care: Certain patients don't sleep well. Others may be apt to wander from the house and are unable to manage themselves properly. Some psychotic patients must be supervised constantly. Doctors and nurses don't work twenty-four-hour days, yet some care givers assume this burden and risk the serious repercussions of care-giver burnout (see Chapter 2).

• heartbreak: Mental anguish is one of the most intense pains imaginable. Sensitive care givers may know when their loved ones are suffering—and this can hurt deeply. Empathic feelings can bond patients and care givers closer together. They can also fill care givers with a profound and very private pain.

• ineffective treatment: Sometimes, especially in the treatment of individuals with severe mental illness, prescribed medication and therapy do not work. Or perhaps they mask some symptoms while bringing others into view. There are many possibilities, each more exasperating than the next. Because of the complicated, sometimes misunderstood nature of mental illness, it may be difficult for the psychiatrist to choose the best medication immediately. Many attempts may be made before the most appropriate type of medication is found. Family support groups have helped many care givers and mentally ill persons cope with this frustrating situation.

• family conflicts: The presence of a mentally ill family member can set off household tensions that lead to family problems. Unfortunately, such family conflicts can also create an atmosphere that may cause relapse in susceptible persons recovering at home.

• the misguided-love cure: Love can be good medicine, but when a loved one has a serious mental illness love alone is not enough. Indeed, some care givers believe that the more love and emotional energy they pour into their relatives the better the chances of recovery. Such efforts can be emotionally depleting to care givers and suffocating to their loved ones.

• legal problems: In some states care givers are faced with exasperating legal dilemmas. Take New York, for example. There a mentally ill person cannot be admitted to a psychiatric hospital for observation and care against his or her wishes. The patient can be hospitalized involuntarily when two physicians or a "commissioner's designee" say that immediate psychiatric hospital care is needed because the individual is a danger to self and/or others. You should know that this is a simplified version of the New York State law, but this and other laws like it are designed to protect patient rights and to prevent indiscriminate hospitalization.

Unfortunately, such laws set up dilemmas for many well-meaning families. For example, what does a family do when a psychotic relative is not a danger to self and/or others, yet is incapable of living alone and is nearly impossible to manage during home care? Furthermore, the ill person may deny that he or she is ill and refuse to be admitted to a psychiatric hospital for treatment and care. Many families in this predicament turn to support groups for advice or foster families who can take the mentally ill person in part-time or full time (see below).

• medication compliance: It is not unusual for a patient to forget or refuse to take prescribed medication. Indeed, this problem plagues many families. Refusing to comply with psychiatrist's orders may be due to a number of things. For example, your relative may be feeling better and not understand the need for continuing the medication. Or he or she may not be able to adhere to a disciplined schedule without help from you or others because of illness. There are many possibilities, but the bottom line is this: To alleviate disturbing symptoms mentally ill individuals must take their medication as prescribed. Contact the physician at the first signs of noncompliance.

• lack of information: Families need information about their relative's mental illness and expectations for recovery, and practical advice to help them cope with difficult behavior. They have a right to expect this from professionals. But the relationship between patient and therapist must be a confidential one and sometimes confidentiality prevents the family from knowing all they want to know. Added to that, some therapists shield their patients behind a cloak of secrecy. Which leads to the question: Does such secrecy protect the patient—or the therapist?

When families can't get the information they need, they are forced to turn elsewhere, such as to books, other mental health professionals, and family support groups.

How You Can Ease the Stress-Makers

Without question you should take time away from the home scene to help alleviate the inevitable stresses of care (see Chapter 2).

• Locate support services by contacting your mental health

association, local agencies, social worker, or family support groups. Delegate patient-care tasks to other family members whenever possible.

• Ask a trusted friend or neighbor to stay with your loved one for a brief time while you catch a movie, go shopping, or join friends for dinner. Churches or synagogues may provide volunteers who can help, too.

• Some communities have "psychosocial clubs" or day-care programs for eligible mentally ill persons. Here, mentally ill individuals socialize with each other, or may receive vocational training in a supervised setting. Some communities have "foster family" programs. Foster families take in the mentally ill on a part-time or full-time basis. This gives the patient's family time to rest and recoup. Foster families receive payment for this service. Consult a social worker for more information or referral.

Family Support Groups

All around the nation support groups for relatives of the mentally ill are springing up. They serve many functions. For instance, they provide information about mental illness, the latest treatments, referrals to reputable professionals, sources of help during crises, community services, and available financial aids. Some of the groups also lobby for patients' rights, work for legislation and funding to ensure quality institutional and community services for the chronically mentally ill, and monitor services being offered. Family support groups help reassure families and let them know they're not alone.

Furthermore, there are groups for the mentally ill themselves. Their goals include providing needed outlets to discuss frustrations and concerns, as well as help prevent relapse.

To find the group that best meets your needs, check out the addresses below:

The National Alliance for the Mentally Ill
1234 Massachusetts Ave., N.W.
Suite 721
Washington, D.C. 20005

This is the parent organization of 177 family support groups that provide families with the help they need to care for loved ones who are mentally ill. Write to locate the support group nearest you.

Reach
c/o The Mental Health Association of Minnesota
5501 Green Valley Dr.
Suite 103
Bloomington, Minn. 55437

Reach is a nationwide program with its national clearinghouse in Minnesota. It is a mutual-help support program for families of the mentally ill. Write for more information and the Reach group nearest you.

Recovery, Inc.
116 S. Michigan Ave.
Chicago, Ill. 60603

Recovery, Inc. is an association of nervous and former mental patients. It promotes a self-help method for the mentally ill. Its goal is to prevent relapse in former mental patients and chronicity in nervous patients. It is operated, managed, supported, and controlled by patients and former patients trained in the recovery method.

More information: There are support groups for patients and or families that specialize in *specific* mental illnesses, such as manic depression and schizophrenia. Contact your local mental health association or social worker for referral.

How to Get Your Loved One on the Road to Recovery

Your loved one may have an easier time regaining control of his or her life if the home scene is relatively stress-free. With this in mind, try to avoid family conflicts. Keep excessive noise and commotion to a minimum, especially during the early weeks of convalescence.

Your family member may or may not have been hospitalized. Regardless, most mentally ill persons recovering at home are not dulled by their illnesses. And they are not immune to the nuances and innuendoes of conversation. Remember, your loved one may have finely tuned antennae that can read true feelings in your eyes, or hear between the pauses of your sentences. He or she may be devastated by any signs of disapproval, embarrassment, or guilt.

Try to act as natural as possible with your loved one. Talk to him or her as you would to any other family member. Don't be oversolicitous or condescending. It may be necessary to adjust your behavior so that your gestures, intonations, and words tell your relative that you are sincerely concerned and are trying to understand what he or she is experiencing.

Overprotectiveness, too, can do more harm than good to your relative. Abraham A. Low, M.D., the late psychiatrist and founder of Recovery, Inc., and a pioneer in the area of family support groups and after-care for the mentally ill, described some of the dangers in his book *Lectures to Relatives of Former Patients.* "The ex-patient is watched, cautioned, superintended, directed, and interfered with. The unceasing supervision suggests to him that the reality of recovery is not trusted—once mentally ill, always mentally ill. The stigma of mental disease rears its ugly head and stares in his perplexed face.

"If the ex-patient rebels, insisting on a measure of free move-

ment and self-directed action, he is likely to be reminded that he
has to 'take it easy,' that he is still 'nervous,' and in need of
'lots of rest.' With subtle reminders of this kind the fact is pain-
fully accentuated that although discharged he is still on probation;
once mentally ill, always mentally ill. The house situation is now
heavy with the spirit of stigma."

To improve the quality of home care for your loved one, note
the following suggestions offered by the Mental Health Association in Suffolk County. This association, based on Long Island,
New York, sponsors a family support group for relatives of the
mentally ill, and has published a helpful guide that provides care
tips and emotional support for families providing home care,
called "'Helping Hands' You Are Not Alone." For a copy write:
The Mental Health Association of Suffolk County, P.O. Box
519, Brentwood, N.Y. 11717. Enclose $2.00. The following is
adapted from it.

• Be prepared for your mentally ill relative to become more
self-sufficient. The goal of treatment is to make emotionally troubled individuals more independent. That may mean taking some
risks. If you don't allow your loved one to take some risks, you
will not allow him or her to succeed.

• Be honest, open, and realistic with your relative and yourself.
You will be able to help your loved one if he or she can trust
you. If you lie or trick your loved one back into treatment you
will destroy trust and your future efforts to help will be met with
doubt. Know that severe mental illness can distort your relative's
view of reality. If you try to hide the truth or trick your loved
one you will only add to his or her confusion. Remember, if your
relative has a distorted sense of reality, you cannot argue with
him or her to change the perception. By the same token, you do
your loved one a disservice by agreeing with him or her. Make
reality available to your relative without forcing the issue.

• Expect that you may be the object of your relative's negative
feelings. Sometimes, when a person works through a problem,

he or she may express anger, depression, guilt, or anxiety. Your loved one may be encouraged by his or her therapist to vent feelings in order to gain relief and achieve insight. Your job (often a difficult one) is to allow your relative to do so. Try not to be dismayed. Your understanding here may be very important to your loved one's progress.

• Be consistent and decisive with your relative, but not inflexible. Your loved one's illness may contribute to his or her indecisiveness or erratic behavior. You can help him or her if you provide a secure living situation, help create a structured environment, and keep your promises and commitments. If you are too inflexible or dominating, you may find yourself in perpetual conflict with your family member. There are times when you must be firm, but mix firmness with gentleness and flexibility.

• Beware of jeopardizing other family relationships and your own emotional health because of your loved one's mental illness. Talk openly with family and trusted friends about what you are going through. Of course, consider joining a family support group so that you may express and share your feelings. Know that you can't help your mentally ill relative if you are not feeling physically and emotionally strong. Be sure to allow time for yourself away from the home-care scene. And seek professional help if you think you need some extra support.

• Be realistic about the professional's ability to help. Do not expect your relative's problems to be resolved quickly. Do not expect mental health professionals to take complete responsibility for your loved one's difficulties. You and your relative retain some responsibility for coping with the situation.

• Request your rights to service in the appropriate way. Always be firm and polite, never arrogant or hostile. You'll get better results. Listen carefully to agency representatives. Chances are they're telling you the truth. There may be no services available to satisfy your need. By the same token, don't be too quick to take no for an answer.

• Know that your relative may change as a result of professional help and treatment. Accept these changes. They may mean that your relationship with your loved one will alter. For instance, one young woman said that her brother had changed after treatment for severe depression. Prior to treatment the ill brother had been quiet and withdrawn. Now, after therapy and medication, he was more talkative and willing to express his feelings. The sister had to adjust to the difference in her brother's behavior.

Your instinct may be to resist changes in your relative, too. If you have questions about your family member's "changes" or you need advice to help you cope, consult the mental health professional.

Compassionate Care Tips for Care Givers

Dealing with a loved one who is mentally ill is never easy and I don't intend to offer you pat answers and fast how-to advice here.

Consider the following information as a supplement to professional advice. Because of space limitations, the guidelines on these next pages are very general. They should not be substituted for specific suggestions made by professionals that are intended to answer your relative's special needs.

Note: If you need additional information; read books and other printed material about your relative's illness. Watch for newspaper listings of mental health programs and lectures. Join a family support group and get involved in a community organization related to mental health.

Anxiety

Anxiety is a type of fear. Mild anxiousness, on occasion, is normal. It's part of our mental and physical alert systems that enable us to anticipate danger and take appropriate action. But severe and recurrent feelings of anxiousness can be part of a stress reaction in a mentally ill person.

What are the signs of anxiety?

Your relative may experience any one or combination of the following: restlessness, dread, loneliness, fear, hostility, increased muscular tension, chest pains, nausea, vomiting, irritability, hypersensitivity to noise and lights.

How can you help?

Stay calm and let your loved one know that you care. He or she may feel better after sharing certain upsetting thoughts or ideas with you. Even if his or her ideas seem silly and unimportant, it's best not to show your reaction to them.

Relaxation techniques may help some people. A warm bath, shower, or light massage may bring relief. Or try to distract your relative with a comforting story, diverting television show, or favorite record.

Let me add that anxiety can make a person feel very isolated. Your family member may be afraid to be left alone. In such cases, stay with your loved one until the anxiety subsides. In fact, the contact of your body (an embrace, hand holding) may be soothing to an anxious person. Remember, though, that some people are not receptive to physical demonstrativeness.

Severe episodes of anxiety that interfere with normal functioning, continue to get worse, and/or last longer require professional attention. A physician or psychiatrist may prescribe medication such as tranquilizers to give your relative relief.

Delusions

Your relative may have delusions. These are false ideas or distortions of reality.

How can you help?

I suggest that you speak to your loved one's therapist to determine the best way for you to cope with his or her delusions. Generally speaking, it's best not to let your relative think that you believe what he says. Try to ignore their content.

Listen carefully to the tone in which a delusion is expressed. This tone may suggest anxiety, concern, etc. Instead of responding to the delusion's story, reach your loved one by saying, "You sound fearful/anxious/concerned, etc. I know that you are having a difficult time."

Speak in specifics to your relative, not in vague generalities. Generalities may be misinterpreted and these can feed delusions.

Remember, too, not to seem secretive with your mentally ill relative. And don't talk about your loved one in his or her presence.

Depression

When we feel depressed we may say we have the blues or feel low. Most often this is a natural reaction to an event in our lives such as a job problem, loss of a loved one, or serious illness. Indeed, for many people depressions are phases that pass relatively quickly. But there are depressions that may be severe and prolonged. They can occur without obvious cause. When these very low moods interfere with everyday functioning, professional help is needed.

What are the signs?
Watch for feelings of sadness, emptiness, low self-esteem, anxiousness, hopelessness, inability to find joy in anything. Physical signs may appear such as stomach problems, racing or palpitating heart beat, sleep disturbances (excessive sleep, early morning wakefulness, difficulty sleeping or staying asleep). Your loved one may display little interest in his or her job, personal appearance, etc.

How can you help?
Try to understand how your relative is feeling. Ask the therapist for guidance. Know that your loved one may be in profound emotional pain. He or she needs to know that you care and are trying to understand. Don't reprimand him or her for not feeling

well. Likewise, asking your patient to "rise above the problem" is pointless, as most severely depressed people cannot help their moods.

Many depressed individuals respond well to antidepressant medication. The physician or psychiatrist may select one from an assortment of possibilities. If medication therapy is chosen, it may take some time to determine the drug that will best help your loved one. In addition, many antidepressants take two to three weeks to work. Other treatments used in severe depression include electroshock therapy. Here, an electric current to the brain induces convulsive seizures that can help alleviate depression in certain patients. Consult the psychiatrist for more information.

Hostile Behavior

Your family member may show anger or threaten harm to you or self.

What are the signs?
Watch for heightened anger, verbal abusiveness, excessive or uncharacteristic use of profanity, insincere sweetness, violent activity.

How can you help?
Hostile behavior is usually a gradual process. It rarely happens suddenly, so you will probably be able to predict what will set your relative off—and may be able to avert that type of activity or language. To help manage a hostile person, consider these suggestions.

• Don't approach the person. Don't reach out. He or she may think that you are going to attack. In response your relative may strike you. On the other hand, you may sense that your loved one needs to be hugged. Perhaps you remember that a warm embrace worked during similar moments in the past. Remember: such a gesture is risky and should be tried with great caution.

• Stay calm. Speak in a well-modulated, nonthreatening voice. If you find that your every action and word seems to increase your relative's hostility, try to leave the scene and then call for help.

• Judge the way to handle your family member based on past experience. Some hostile individuals can be diverted if you suggest another activity such as television watching or music listening. Some respond if they are told to go to another room to cool off. Clearly, each case is different. Consult the mental health professionals if you have any questions.

• Don't challenge your relative. Furthermore, if your loved one has a weapon, don't try to disarm him or her.

• If you sense that you are in danger, leave the room at once. Do not, however, turn your back abruptly on your relative, as this may provoke him or her.

• Protect yourself and other members of your family by removing all weapons from the house. Try to understand what triggers your relative's attacks of hostility and see to it that such provocation is kept to an absolute minimum.

• Persistent hostile behavior demands medical evaluation.

Manic Depression

There are variations on the theme of manic depressive illness. Generally, it's recognized by exaggerated mood swings that move from normal to elation or to depression, or alternating. The illness may subside only to recur sometime later. The severity of it varies, and not all manic depressives have the classic mood swings.

It's worth noting that the first manic episode rarely occurs before late adolescence, and may not show until the late twenties, thirties, or even later. Until you see the first manic attack you may have a tough time believing your relative capable of one.

What are the signs?
The manic side of your relative's illness may emerge as elation, irritability, overtalkativeness, flight of ideas, and/or increased

physical activity where the individual appears to be in constant movement. Know that moods of elation may not be joyous as much as frenzied. Indeed, your relative may seem to be battling depression even in the midst of an elated mood. Not long after an upswing of elation, your loved one may crash into a severe depression. Know, too, that some individuals become overindulgent during the manic phase. For example, your loved one may go on shopping sprees, make reckless investments, and so on.

The depressive part of this illness may leave your relative in despair. He or she may display the classic signs of depression after a manic attack. However, there are some who are called manic depressives who show the depressive side of the illness but without the "highs" associated with the manic phase.

The scenario for a manic attack differs among individuals. Generally, your relative may seem odd before the episode goes into full swing. He or she may act inappropriately or recklessly. Your loved one may have unexpected outbursts and/or display increased physical activity. As the mania overpowers he or she may undergo mood changes that bounce back between elation and anger.

Tip: You may be able to anticipate your relative's manic attack by noting his or her response to criticism. If your criticism sparks an inappropriate outburst of anger, it can be a strong sign that a manic episode is on the way. Seek professional guidance.

Some good news: Many manic depressives have been helped by a drug called lithium. This medication controls manic and depressive episodes in receptive individuals. Indeed, many manic depressives can lead normal lives when they take their lithium doses daily and have their blood lithium levels checked regularly. Blood level checks are important because too little lithium is ineffective and too much can be toxic, and in some cases fatal. Be sure that your loved one is being treated by a psychiatrist who is highly qualified and experienced in monitoring lithium levels in manic depressives.

Schizophrenia

Schizophrenia is an illness that often runs in families. It rarely appears in childhood; usually it emerges when a person is in his or her twenties. The illness is triggered when the susceptible person is under stress. Schizophrenia may appear in the form of an episode.

The typical way an episode is recognized is when the patient experiences strange notions. For example, your loved one may think that he or she is hearing, smelling, or seeing things that are not real. These are called hallucinations. He or she may believe things that are not true, as with delusions.

Some schizophrenics believe that others are out to get them (paranoid schizophrenia); that others can read their thoughts; or that they are getting special messages from external agents such as the television or radio. Some schizophrenics believe they are famous people or that they can see into the future.

These disturbances of thought, feeling, and behavior vary from patient to patient and may be changed by time.

What are the signs?

Your relative may experience any one or more of the following: hallucinations, delusions, disorganized thinking, uncontrollable rushes of thought, anxiety, disturbances of feeling (laughs at sad things, cries at lighter moments); talking to oneself, difficulty focusing attention, absorption in a private world, and using a private language are other signs.

How can you help?

Consider the atmosphere in your home. According to a recent study at the School of Medicine of the University of Southern California, the average home life is too stressful for most schizophrenics to tolerate. However, if families learn to cope with their problems, schizophrenics improve dramatically.

Family stress-relieving techniques can be learned. If your

household atmosphere is a tense one, call a mental health professional to find out how you can ease the stresses in your home.

Encourage your loved one to get at least seven hours of sleep
to help keep stress from mounting up and causing problems.

Know that there are certain substances your ill relative should
avoid as they can provoke a schizophrenic episode in susceptible
persons: coffee, cigarettes, and other common stimulants; nasal
decongestants have been found to contain ingredients that can
trigger an attack. Hallucinogens such as LSD and PCP (angel
dust) can cause trouble. So can amphetamines (diet pills, uppers,
etc.), marijuana, and heavy use of alcohol. Moderate use of
alcohol may not cause trouble, but check with the psychiatrist to
be sure.

Understand that hallucinations may be part of your loved one's
illness and that these episodes are out of his or her control. Don't
reject the hallucinations. On the other hand, don't act as if they
are real. You might say, for example, "What was the odor you
say you smelled like?" This type of comment acknowledges the
hallucination, but does not make it seem very credible.

Know that what you say and do can influence your loved one.
Indeed, he or she may not respond, but may be affected nonetheless. For example, at times your family member may seem to
be in another world. You may be tempted to talk about your
relative as if he or she were not there. This is not wise, as your
words may register.

Mental health professionals can show you ways to communicate more effectively with your relative. You may also need
professional advice when you try to teach your loved one skills
so that he or she can become more self-sufficient. One psychiatric
social worker suggested care givers begin by teaching their relatives to do simple household tasks such as laundry or house
cleaning (his or her own room, etc.). "Try the reward system,"
suggested a psychiatric social worker. "Every time the mentally
ill person learns a task or another step in performing the task he
or she can be given a treat, money, or time with the care giver

alone." Furthermore, a professional can help you set up behavior modification techniques so that you can reinforce wanted behavior and undermine unwanted behavior.

Try to appreciate your loved one's progress, no matter how small the steps may seem. The schizophrenic's world can be a frightening one. Your relative may experience disorienting hallucinations or anxiety-provoking delusions. Try to empathize with these feelings and let your loved one know that you are concerned and supportive, loving but not overprotective.

How disabled will your relative be? Of course, each case is different. The easier it is to control the schizophrenia, the less disabled he or she will be. Medication is of major importance in the control of this illness. Most schizophrenics must continue on maintenance medications to keep their symptoms under control.

Some schizophrenics give up and let the illness take over. Others try to live with and in spite of their condition. Still others are able to resume jobs and activities once symptoms are managed properly. Naturally, there are jobs that are not easy for schizophrenics to handle. Vocational rehabilitation may be needed to help your loved one lead a productive life. Consult a social worker for more information.

One final word—relapses: Know how to spot the early warning signs so that you can get help for your loved one as soon as possible. One early signal is sleeplessness. If your relative cannot sleep two nights in a row, call his or her psychiatrist. Another sign: If your relative has experienced hallucinations or delusions relapses in many cases start the same way. So if your patient has already had one, watch for similar relapse signals next time.

Medication

I suggest that you learn as much as you can about the medication prescribed for your loved one. Each type may have side effects in addition to expected benefits.

Use the following abbreviated list as a guide only. Check with the physician or psychiatrist for complete information about medication prescribed for your relative.

Drug type: antianxiety drugs (Ativan, Librium, Serax, Valium).

Dangerous interactions: no alcohol. Do not use when working machinery. Do not take with MAO inhibitors and central nervous system depressants.

Typical side effects: drowsiness, fatigue, slurred speech, diminished muscle control, sleep difficulties.

Drug type: antipsychotics (Compazine, Haldol, Mellaril, Navane, Stelazine, Thorazine); prescribed to manage psychotic disorders.

Dangerous interactions: should not be used in patients who are severely depressed or comatose, or who have major cardiovascular or liver disease; should not be taken if patient is already receiving large amounts of hypnotics. Avoid hazardous machinery.

Typical side effects: blurred vision, drowsiness, ejaculatory problems, tardive dyskinesia (see below), dry mouth, restlessness (especially Stelazine), lower convulsive threshold (especially Thorazine).

Drug type: barbiturates, hypnotics (Dalmane, Doriden, Methaqualone, Placidyl, Seconal); prescribed to bring about sleep.

Dangerous interactions: patients who are hypersensitive to sedatives, severely depressed, suicidal; no alcohol and other central nervous system depressants. Avoid hazardous machinery.

Typical side effects: addiction, drowsiness, mild gastric discomfort, headache, disorientation.

Drug type: monoamine oxidase inhibitors (MAO inhibitors, such as Nardil, Parnate); prescribed for reactive depression.

Dangerous interactions: Certain patients should be very cautious such as those with cardiovascular disease, diabetes, or epilepsy. Avoid taking or eating the following: Lomotil, alcohol, avocadoes, aged cheese, Bovril, Marmite, soy sauce, wild game, bananas, canned figs, Chianti wine, chocolate, chicken livers, licorice, meat extracts and tenderizers, pickled/kippered herring, pineapple, raisins, raw yeast, sour cream, yogurt, nasal and pulmonary decongestants, sleeping or antiappetite medications and antidepressants. Mixing any of the previous substances with MAO inhibitors can lead to exceedingly elevated blood pressure causing stroke or death.

Typical side effects: insomnia, urinating problems, dizziness, tremors, fatigue.

Drug type: tricyclic antidepressants (Adapin, Elavil, Norpramin, Pertofrane, Sinequan, Tofranil); prescribed to treat depression and anxiety.

Dangerous interactions: Do not give to patients with glaucoma or urinary retention or those with heart disease, angina conditions, or active seizure disorders; no alcohol, MAO inhibitors; no Elavil and Placidyl combinations.

Typical side effects: dry mouth, blurred vision, mild tremor, hypotension, insomnia, skin eruptions, nightmares.

Tardive dyskinesia can occur when a patient has been on high doses of anti-psychotic medications for a long time. The signs of tardive dyskinesia are involuntary rhythmic movements of the face, tongue, or, less often, other muscles; protrusion of the tongue, puffing of the cheeks or jaw, puckering of the mouth, chewing movements, involuntary movements of arms and legs. If medication is stopped in time, many of the symptoms of tardive dyskinesia can be reversed.

Your relative should be monitored carefully by medical professionals if he or she is taking any of the anti-psychotics.

For additional information you may find any of the following helpful.

The American Psychiatric Association
See Chapter 14.

E. R. Squibb & Sons, Inc.
P.O. Box 4000
Princeton, N.J. 08540

Write for their pamphlet, *Living with Schizophrenia.*

Neurotics Anonymous
P.O. Box 4866
Cleveland Park Station
Washington, D.C. 20008

This organization offers a twelve-step plan to help persons recovering from mental illness stay well.

Alcoholics Anonymous
P.O. Box 459
Grand Central Station
New York N.Y. 10017

The National Self-help Clearinghouse
CUNY Rm. 1225
133 West 42nd St.
New York, N.Y. 10036

12

Loving Home Care for the Older Adult

Many elderly people prefer the privacy and independence of living alone, but there are times when this just isn't possible. The illnesses and disabilities that may come with aging can force an elderly person to turn to others for help. In the great majority of cases, assistance is provided by the family.

If you are the relative or friend of an older adult, you may be involved in one of several home-care styles.

• You may keep in touch with an elderly relative who is staying in his or her home with the aid of home-health professionals and other support services.

• You may move your loved one into your home and use the services available in your community.

• You may investigate semi-independent living arrangements for the elderly, such as congregate housing where modest assistance for residents is provided, such as meal programs, health care, and social activities.

• You may look toward a nursing home as the best care choice for your loved one when home care is no longer fitting.

This chapter is designed to give you a clearer understanding of the home-care possibilities for older adults. Here, too, you will learn practical care tips to enable you to give quality care in an empathetic and compassionate way.

Beware of Dangerous Stereotypes

More Americans are living to ripe old ages than ever before. We can thank improved environmental conditions, better nutrition, and the wonders of medical science. Tied to this perk from progress is this fact: The longer we live, the more we are prone to the physical effects of aging. Of course, I mean the proverbial gray hair, wrinkles—and changes inside the body.

Unfortunately, these changes feed treacherous stereotypes. Many of us come to specific—and frequently wrong—conclusions about the older adults we see. We doubt their productivity and creativity. We may question their abilities to learn new skills. We may say that old people are inflexible, eccentric, slow moving, and dim witted. One man told me that he thought all old people looked alike.

Without question, these stereotypes deny older adults their individuality and worth. Frankly, all people do not age in the same way or at the same pace. Indeed, most of the elderly remain throughout life as intelligent as they ever were.

Yes, there are older adults who use their age and weaknesses as an excuse for dependency; but there are many more who overcome their deficiencies and play up their strengths.

My point: When you, the care giver, provide care for your older relative, take time to see that relative as an individual— not as an old person. This is the first step toward bringing enhanced feeling and insight to your role as care giver. And the more in touch you are with your loved one's emotional and physical needs, the easier it will be for you to accept and relate to your elderly relative during care.

Aging: Changes for You to Consider

Take a moment to read the abbreviated list below. It will help you step into your loved one's emotional and physical shoes:

On the physical side, your loved one may be:
• experiencing diminishing muscle strength, coordination, and balance
• trying to adjust to body changes that create a new self-image
• having infrequent moments of forgetfulness (research suggests not due to loss of memory but due to a slowing down in the retrieval of information)
• dealing with senses that may be less precise (taste, smell, sight, touch, hearing)
• becoming tired more easily
• having poorer circulation
• noticing dry skin and diminishing skin elasticity
• having a bit of difficulty adjusting to temperature changes
• fearful of falls as bones become less tensile and breaks happen more easily.

On the emotional side, your loved one may be:
• fearful about loss of independence
• worried about diminishing financial resources
• apprehensive about retirement
• overwhelmed by personal losses (death of spouse, friends, relatives, moving away from own home or neighborhood)
• fearful of illness and death.

What is it like to grow older? The above is a mini-preview of the inevitable changes we must all face. Broaden your understanding of your elderly loved one by reading as much as you can about aging. Let me suggest some books to get your started: *A Good Age*, by Alex Comfort, Crown Publishers, New York, 1976; *Fact Book on Aging*, National Council on Aging, Washington, D.C., 1977; *When Your Parents Grow Old*, by Jane Otten and Florence Shelley, Signet Books, New York, 1978; *Why Survive? Being Old in America*, by Robert Butler, M.D., Harper & Row, New York, 1975; *You and Your Aging Parent*, by Barbara Silverstone and Helen Hyman, Pantheon, New York, 1982.

When Is a Nursing Home the Right Choice?

Nursing homes are patient-care facilities that, ideally, provide an acceptable place for older adults to live. Consider a nursing home instead of home care when your elderly relative needs supervision twenty-four hours a day. If, however, your relative needs a less restrictive and less intensive type of care, try to arrange for a combination of services and/or programs that may be more appropriate than the nursing home alternative (more on that later).

What types of services do nursing homes offer? Clearly, this depends on the type of home you're talking about. Generally speaking, nursing home services can include nutritious meals, medical care, personal care assistance, rehabilitation therapy, social activities, and the companionship of others. Some are geared more toward personal care. Others cater to medical needs. And there are those that are somewhere in between.

The specific types of homes that exist fall into a number of categories. To find out which types are in your area consult your patient's physician, geriatric social worker affiliated with county social services, area agency on aging, local or state health department, hospital social services department, church groups, or the Yellow Pages of your phone book. Beware, though, of enticing advertisements. The quality of a home is not measured by the cleverness of an ad, but by its adherence to established regulations and the quality of its services. You will have to do some homework to find the facility worthy of your loved one.

As for the types of homes, know that two kinds have been defined by Medicare and Medicaid: skilled nursing facilities (SNF) and intermediate care facilities (ICF).

The SNF is a nursing home that has been certified as meeting federal standards within the Social Security Act. Broadly speaking, the SNF offers skilled nursing care for patients recuperating from surgery or illness and those with long-term conditions. This type of home is similar to a hospital as it provides twenty-four-

hour nursing services along with medical supervision and rehabilitation programs.

The ICF is also certified and abides by federal standards. However, this home offers less complete health care and similar services than the SNF. The older adults who live in ICF's are people
unable to live alone, yet are not disabled enough to require twenty-
four-hour nursing care. These homes highlight personal care and
social services.

Know, too, that nursing homes fall into profit (proprietary)
and nonprofit (nonproprietary) categories. Most often church,
ethnic, state, county, or charitable homes or homes run by government agencies at federal, state, or local levels are nonprofit.
Many of these residences have superior reputations. Nursing homes
that are part of a chain are usually proprietary homes.

Nursing-home selection should be done with care. It should
be made in collaboration with medical professionals and, whenever possible, the elderly patient. To learn more about nursing
homes write for the free government booklet, *How to Select a
Nursing Home*, the U.S. Department of Health and Human Services, Health Care Financing Administration, Division of Long-
Term Care, Baltimore, Md. 21207. It will answer many of your
questions.

Tip: The law says that each state must have a state nursing
home ombudsman. The ombudsman is concerned with problems
that affect residents of nursing homes such as safety, welfare,
and rights. Consider contacting your state ombudsman to determine if there are any serious complaints about the nursing home
you may be deciding on. For the address in your state write: the
United States Administration on Aging, 330 Independence Ave.,
S.W., Washington, D.C. 20201, att: Staff for Nursing Home
Interests.

What Kind of Nursing Home
Does Your Relative Need?

To know this, speak to your loved one's personal physician to determine the most suitable level of care and whether or not special services must be provided at the selected facility. Remember, too, that location should be a significant factor when deciding on a home. The residence should be in an area pleasing to your relative, it should be close enough to family and friends, and it should be near a hospital providing emergency health-care services. It is possible that the homes in your immediate area will not meet your loved one's needs. In such cases it may be wise to consider establishments outside the immediate area.

Beware of Nursing Home Phobia

Recently an editor at a well-known gerontology publication told me the story of an eighty-four-year-old nursing home resident. He was placed in a skilled nursing facility to convalesce after a double hernia operation. He did well in the hospital, but upon arrival at the nursing home and during the couple of weeks that followed he became so emotionally distraught that he was impossible to handle.

The elderly man was sent back to the hospital for a re-evaluation. There, it was discovered that he was terrified of nursing homes. He feared abuse, tainted food, and poor care. Indeed, his preconceived notion of nursing home life was so horrendous that he became hysterical within its walls. In time the hospital staff persuaded him that his fears were unjustified. They encouraged him to try the nursing home again. On the second time around he did just fine.

This eighty-four-year-old man isn't alone in his nursing home phobia. You, too, may believe that nursing homes are repulsive places that mistreat the elderly. In fact, you may be feeling very guilty about placing your loved one in a home because of the terrible stories you have heard.

Yes, there have been nursing homes where patient care was appalling and the facilities weren't fit for human beings. I don't doubt that squalid homes still exist. However, there *are* many homes that employ highly trained staffs ready to meet the medical, social, and emotional needs of each patient, homes that provide a pleasant atmosphere and competent care.

My point: A high-quality certified home may be the best choice in certain circumstances. Learn more about the types of nursing homes and services offered. A little knowledge can dispel your worst fears—and help you locate a facility, if necessary, that provides compassionate, top-quality care.

A Checklist to Help You Find a Top-Quality Nursing Home

Use the seven "don'ts" that follow as guidelines to get you started. There are many things to consider when deciding on a nursing home. Your loved one's physician or a social worker can offer further help.

• Don't tolerate unsanitary conditions. Beware of unpleasant smells (urine, garbage, etc.), flies, roaches, dirty floors/bathrooms and eating areas, untidy living quarters. Insist on automatic dishwasher for all dishes, sterilized bedpans, urinals, medical equipment.

• Don't accept poor-quality health services. Beware of staff shortages, unqualified employees, indifferent care. Know the qualifications of the nursing home physician and his availability to the patients.

• Don't tolerate low-grade food services. Watch out for little variety to menus, lack of fruits, vegetables, and well-balanced meals. Be sure special diets are adhered to, that the kitchen staff is well organized and sanitary. Sample the food yourself. Is it good? Would you want to eat it every day? Are adequate portions served?

• Don't accept unsafe or overcrowded conditions. Be sure there are proper exits, functional exit doors, smoke detectors, operable sprinkler systems. Make certain living quarters are comfortable; residents have plenty of space: rooms are well lighted.

• Don't accept inadequate therapy facilities. Depending on your loved one's needs, be sure there are qualified and caring physical, occupational, respiratory, speech, and hearing therapists. Is there private or group counseling for patients who may need it?

• Don't tolerate exorbitant fees. Be wary if you are asked to pay additional fees unless given an adequate and reasonable explanation. Call the welfare authorities if you believe you are being unfairly charged.

• Don't consider a home that does not adequately protect your loved one's possessions or money or a home that does not have a current license. Occasionally, a license will have lapsed, but the home does not reveal this fact to residents and their families—watch out!

Your Home-Care Strategy

Once your elderly relative can no longer live independently, you'll have to decide about other provisions for care. Sometimes this decision must be made in the midst of a health crisis—often after an older adult has been hospitalized for a serious illness or surgery. Sometimes it comes more gradually, the natural result of a long, disabling condition.

Once you realize that a care change is needed, you and, whenever possible, your elderly relative should decide what it will be. Assuming that you've ruled out the nursing home alternative, you are left with a mix of choices. Your loved one, if appropriate, may receive care in his or her own home, your home, or some other housing arrangement (congregate housing, sheltered housing, etc.). To help you figure out the best and most humane possibility, fill out the Care Strategy Questionnaire below. Having all the facts in front of you may help crystallize your own and your relative's decision:

Care-Strategy Questionnaire

• What is your relative's current mental condition?

• What is the status of your relative's physical health?

• If there are mental and/or physical problems is improvement possible? What must be done to facilitate improvement?

• How much nursing care, if any, is needed?

• Are any rehabilitative services (physical, speech, occupational therapy) needed?

• Where does your loved one prefer to have care administered?

• What is the extent of your relative's financial resources? Insurance coverage? How much financial help can you or other family members give?

• What are the local home-health care services available to help your relative?

• What other supervised housing alternatives are available?

• Who can help supervise your loved one's care, if necessary? Your relative? You? Other members of the family? In-home health-service providers (visiting nurse service, etc.)?

Professionals can help you answer these questions and develop a suitable strategy for care: The physician, for example, can clarify your loved one's medical needs. The nurse can make suggestions about the older adult's nursing needs. A social worker can assess community services and how they may come to your loved one's aid. You can also determine what local services are available by contacting your local or state area agency on aging and by checking the phone book.

One last important point. Encourage your relative to express his or her wishes and then be sensitive to them. Some older adults warm to the idea of moving in with their families. Others reject it vehemently. Still, some will be unable to participate in a decision because of illness or disability. And don't forget about other experts and the help they can provide: therapists, psychologists, and pharmacists can cite "musts" needed to maintain or restore your relative's health.

The bottom line here is team work. It's not necessary for you to go the home-care adventure alone. A care plan can be created with professionals that can dramatically improve the efficiency and caliber of care.

Your Home for Care? What Are You Getting Into?

The move to give home care to an elderly relative can be perilous for you. You may find that your loved one needs you when your own life is brimming with responsibilities to your family or job. Moreover, a new addition to your household may be unsettling, even traumatic, for certain members of the family.

Furthermore, once you've decided to take in an older adult you will be faced with the physical, emotional, and financial demands of care. The more consuming these demands are for you, the more your stress load will increase. Consequently, you may think thoughts and harbor wishes that make you feel guilty and ashamed. You may want to run away from home care or wish your relative would leave. You may secretly investigate other care alternatives—and berate yourself for doing so. These are normal feelings that spring from the pressures of care. And it's no wonder—you must face the implications of your relative's condition and at the same time cope with so many demands.

Perilousness doesn't end here. You may be concerned, even heartbroken, about the changes in your older relative. Of course, you have always known him or her to be a certain way. Now, illness may be causing temporary or permanent changes. As one daughter said, "Can you imagine your mother being an active woman all her life and seeing her slowly deteriorate—wouldn't it affect you?"

Of course it would, and the degree to which you are affected by your loved one's condition will depend on the severity of his or her illness and your own sensitivity.

No matter how well meaning your intentions or how profound your love, stresses, heartache, and frustrations are likely companions to care. You may run into danger if you surpress your feelings. You may, for example, explode with verbal threats you'll live to regret, become indifferent to your elderly relative, or, in extreme situations, cause him or her harm. The key is to head off problems before they occur—and to have the courage to change your care strategy if it is not working for you and/or your loved one. Spot the early warning signs of trouble that may be affecting you: persistent irritability, frequent temper flare-ups, marital problems that intensify or emerge after your relative's arrival, sleep problems (insomnia), sexual difficulties, weight loss, depression, anxiety, diminishing social life and contacts with friends, resentment toward your elderly relative. Be alert to difficulties other family members may be having. Children may have trouble adjusting to your older adult's presence. This can be reflected in learning difficulties, lower grades, hostility toward the elderly relative, and other behavior changes.

My advice to help alleviate the strains of care: Lighten your tensions by talking about them. Friends, family, and professionals can help. A social worker or nurse who is experienced in geriatric care and services can prove invaluable. Contact your local hospital, physician, or county social services department for referrals. Consider support and self-help groups, too.

Let us step beyond home care's hazards. Indeed, there are many joys and rewards that make it all worthwhile. Your home can give your older relative a stable environment that radiates caring, warmth, and love. There, your loved one can maintain the identity and individuality so often lost in the shuffle of institutional settings. Family interaction and activities help keep the elderly mind spry and spirited. As Robin Marantz Henig points out in *The Myth of Senility* (New York: Anchor Press, 1981), "an old mind is like an old muscle. It must be used and challenged to function well. If housed within four empty walls and left to wither the mind will indeed atrophy, roaming back to the past when it was put to good use and unable to snap back into the dreary present even when called upon to do so."

Your elderly relative can also make contributions to you and your family. When appropriate, he or she can share in decision-making and household tasks. And your loved one can keep you in touch with the natural cycles of life. After all, we must all grow older. Better to embrace the realities of aging than deny the inevitable.

Your home for care? There's no question that you may be embarking on a demanding adventure. Yet the frustrations and difficulties may be mitigated by the exquisite emotional bonding that can take place—between you, your family, and your older relative.

Home-Care Helpers

Home care for older adults is made possible by many programs and services offered in communities around the country. Here's a rundown for you to check out. Note that not all home-care helpers suggested here exist in every community. Find out what's available in your area. In addition to ideas about getting the advice you need, already discussed in this chapter, the following can help you tune into the facilities, programs, and services available in your community:

• social services office of the community public welfare agency
• social worker in the hospital where your relative is known
• information and referral services in your community—(not uniformly available throughout the country)
• your state welfare office
• your area or state office on aging (most often in your state's capital or major city).

Adult Day Care

There are two types of programs available in many areas around the nation: the multipurpose type of program and the day hospital program.

The day hospitals are usually attached to health care institutions and receive their patients from them. They have a strong emphasis on health care, physical rehabilitation, and treatment. Multipurpose programs frequently do not provide rehabilitative care and focus instead on patients who are less hampered by illness and have a strong need for social interaction and activities.

According to the National Center for Health Services Research, day care is defined as a program of services provided under professional leadership in an ambulatory care setting for adults who do not need round-the-clock institutional care and yet, because of physical or mental impairments, are not able to assume full-time independent living. Older adults are referred to the programs by their attending physician or other source such as hospital discharge planning program, social service agency, etc. Adult day care tries to maintain and restore a patient's health. Know, too, that there is a social side to many of these programs. Among the services that may be provided, depending on the particular center, are nursing, social services, personal care, meals, transportation, physical occupational therapy, speech therapy, eye examinations, podiatry, and patient activities.

To locate the centers nearest you, write for the *Directory of Adult Day Care Centers* to the U.S. Department of Health and Human Services, Health Care Financing Administration, Health Standards and Quality Bureau, 1849 Gwynn Oak Ave., Baltimore, Md. 21207.

Food Services

Home-delivered meals may be provided to serve nutritious food to older adults in their homes when they are unable to prepare their own. One or two meals may be offered. However, there are programs in some areas that provide five meals a week; a few serve on weekends. In certain areas this program is called Meals-on-Wheels.

Additionally, there are places such as senior citizen centers and schools which serve noon meals. In some places social activities are provided along with food service. In addition to contacting the standard sources of information for the elderly already mentioned, try religious organizations such as Catholic charities, as they sometimes sponsor food services for the elderly.

Foster Homes for Adults

When an elderly person is unable to live alone and he or she prefers not to live with family or the family is unavailable, the foster home may be an alternative. Host families are matched to older persons in the hope of providing living quarters, meals, and security in nice environments.

Fees for this service vary. Some states have programs that pay foster families for giving care. Contact a social worker at your county social service agency to find out if foster homes exist in your area. Only use the services of those known to be reputable and high quality.

Home-Chore Services

Sometimes older adults living alone need some help with household tasks such as cleaning, laundry, snow shoveling, yard maintenance, etc. The Visiting Nurse Service and other organizations supplying homemakers and home-health aides may provide assistance. Check phone book for local addresses. Know, too, that there are often volunteers affiliated with churches or synagogues who may lend a helping hand. Call your local church or synagogue and ask if such individuals are available. Along these lines, try local high-school community service groups for volunteer help, too.

Home-Health Care

See Chapter 2, where the wide variety of health services that can be brought into the home is discussed. An older adult may benefit from in-home services such as visiting nurses, home-health aides, therapists, nutrition counseling, etc. Besides that, medical supplies and assistive devices may be used at home to enable your loved one to avoid hospitalization or a nursing home.

Multigeneration communes

Under one roof, perhaps inside a house or apartment, may live a group of people who range in age from young adult to older adult. One such commune was founded in Boston in 1978 by the Back Bay Aging Concerns Committee. This living arrangement exposes elderly participants to the realities of many generations living together, unlike age-segregated housing.

Protective Services

When an older adult has trouble managing his or her own affairs, protective services may be needed. The goal of this program is to provide financial and legal services to help older adults protect themselves from injury and exploitation. For more information contact your social worker or county social services office.

Special Housing Arrangements

Separate facilities are available in many communities for older or handicapped people. Many are geared to individuals with low or moderate incomes. Some offer social and/or health services to their residents. Among the choices: *Sheltered housing* is designed for people with significant disabilities such as those who are temporarily or permanently impaired (physically or mentally), or frail elderly people who are unable to manage a semiindependent life-style without support services; *congregate housing* is a shared living style for older adults who are still relatively independent but need some help in one or more areas of daily living. Some arrangements furnish central dining, health services, delivery of meals to those unable to take part in group services, housekeeping, recreation, social activities, and/or linen services.

Rent is usually based on the older adult's ability to pay. For more information contact your local area agency on aging or social worker affiliated with county social services.

Telephone Reassurance Programs

Living alone can be very isolating, at times frightening to an elderly person. "Telephone Reassurance" supplies a daily contact for elderly people who live by themselves and are concerned about their safety, security, or have chronic health conditions. Phone calls are arranged for predesignated times. If there is no answer when the volunteer calls, other phone calls are made to neighbors or police to check on the older adult's well-being. For more details about reassurance services in your area, contact your local area agency on aging or senior citizen centers. Also, churches and synagogues may have volunteers who call elderly people to whom they have been assigned.

Along these lines, there are also "beepers," small, portable machines that can be worn by an older adult. In the event of an emergency such as a fall or health crisis when the elderly person cannot get to the phone, the beeper is turned on and signals help. For more information check the Yellow Pages under "Paging and Signaling Services."

Transportation and Escort Services

Many older adults don't have their own transportation to get to health services, shopping centers, and the like. Here, volunteer driver programs or special minibus services for elderly or handicapped people are available. In addition, volunteers may help the elderly by escorting them to and from appointments and other activities. Contact local senior citizen centers, social worker affiliated with county social services, and churches and synagogues that have volunteer groups which may be able to help. There are also services for which you can pay to hire a home attendant or companion to escort the older adult to and from appointments and errands. See Yellow Pages.

Volunteer Visitors

Many volunteers around the country visit home-bound elderly people regularly. This service is especially important to those who do not have regular contact with family or neighbors. Volunteers give companionship, handle some household tasks, escort the elderly to certain activities. Call church groups, synagogues, or county social services for details about volunteer programs in your area.

Your Patient Care Guide

The first six chapters of this book will give you the general information you need to administer top-notch home care. Of course, elderly individuals have additional health problems that are not as prevalent in other age groups. Let the following care tips support the professional advice that you receive from your loved one's physician, nurse, or therapist.

Safety: Is Your Home Older-Adult-Proof?

You've probably heard that falls can be exceedingly dangerous to an elderly person. Indeed, even a slight fall can lead to a serious bone fracture in susceptible patients. That's why you'll want to be alert to hazards that can cause accidents in your home.

• Watch out for unmended shoes, untied shoelaces and loose slippers.

• Check for slippery floor surfaces and scatter rugs.

• Eliminate long electric cords on the floor.

• Be sure all areas of the house or apartment are well lit, especially the stairways.

- Beware of toys and pets underfoot.
- Close open doors (closets, cupboards) and open drawers.
- Make sure floors are dry, that anything spilled is wiped up quickly.

There are also special assistive devices that can be added to your home and/or to your elderly relative's living area that can make movement easier and safer. See Chapter 3 for suggestions and suppliers of aids such as grab bars near the tub and shower, tub and shower chairs, elevated toilet seats, side rails on the bed to prevent falling, wheelchairs, walkers, canes, ramps, and so on.

Also, be prepared for possible emergencies. Check out Chapter 10 to see how to handle the most common ones. Ask the physician about the health crises that can be anticipated and planned for in your relative's case. Fire, too, can be particularly dangerous to older adults confined to wheelchairs or bed. Do you know how to transport your loved one to safety in such situations? Ask the physician or contact your local fire department for advice.

Appetite

As you know, a well-balanced diet is essential to maintain your elderly relative's health. Unfortunately, there are "appetite saboteurs" that prey on elderly appetites. Head them off before they become serious enough to interfere with your loved one's ability to eat properly.

- Chewing troubles can turn eating into a chore rather than a pleasure. Be sure your relative receives regular dental care. False teeth may be needed, or if your relative already has them, repairs may be in order. Jaw difficulties can inhibit ability to open the mouth properly. Arthritis may be the cause. Seek medical evaluation. Also, some older adults may complain of a foul taste in their mouths. Be sure your loved one follows proper mouth hygiene before meals to prevent this problem.
- Poor appetite may be due to many things, from physical illness to emotional distress. Loss of appetite that leads to weight

loss should be discussed with the physician. There are times, however, when weight loss is due to changes in the stomach and bowels because of the aging process. This may be perfectly normal. For example, the stomach may not hold as much as it used to. Digestion may not be as smooth as in younger years. Tip: Your relative may prefer to eat several small meals and a bedtime snack instead of the standard three squares a day.

Arthritis

There are many kinds of arthritis caused by a variety of problems. That is why it's important for your elderly relative to get proper medical evaluation to pinpoint the cause. The two most common types are osteoarthritis and rheumatoid arthritis. *Osteoarthritis* is the most common. Simply, it's the wearing down of joint cartilage, eventually leading to exposure of the underlying bone. Bone then takes the place of the soft cartilage, and the result is that the joints become enlarged and rigid. Osteoarthritis does not cause general symptoms.

Patient complaints

Your relative may say that he or she has joint pain, swelling, and/or stiffness. Disability can occur when the disease strikes knees, hips, and spine.

Treatment

There is no cure. Yet many cases are readily controlled by simple means such as exercise, physical treatments (paraffin baths, moist heat applications, exercise, aspirin, and other medication) Many physicians recommend weight loss in overweight patients to relieve strain on the back, hips, knees, and/or feet. Rest also is very important, as is a well-balanced diet and, when needed, physical therapy.

Watch out for quacks who prescribe all sorts of arthritis cures. This is a chronic disease that can usually be controlled with *proper* medical treatment. Consult the physician or a rheumatologist (a physician who specializes in the diagnosis and treatment of arthritis).

Care tips

Here are some "do's" to bear in mind when caring for your arthritic patient.

• Make sure your patient stays as active as his or her condition allows. Inactivity can cause muscle weakness and additional deformities.

• Remember that your patient may experience some early morning stiffness. In general, osteoarthritis sufferers feel more discomfort with more activity of the affected joints. However, it's important that your loved one follow the right kind of exercise regimen to keep in optimum health. Ask the physician to prescribe a routine appropriate to your patient's condition. In some cases physical therapy is needed for a patient to maintain the full range of motion.

• Remember that your loved one will have good and bad days. Be patient.

• Tell your patient not to hold one position for too long.

• Ask the physician about aspirin and other medications to relieve your patient's discomforts. Watch out for aspirin side effects. There are times, for instance, when large doses of aspirin can cause stomach bleeding. Bloody or very dark stools may clue you into the problem. Other effects to watch for: ringing in the ears and hearing loss.

• Consider assistive devices to make your elderly relative's life easier. Utensils that are built up may be easier for your patient to grasp (forks, knives, spoons, toothbrushes, shaving equipment). Consult an occupational therapist or check out the assistive devices in the catalogues mentioned in Chapter 3 for additional ideas.

Rheumatoid arthritis is an inflammation of the tissue linings of the joints. Eventually, if the patient fails to get proper treatment, the affected joint may become permanently stiffened. The result: pain, muscle spasm, and deformities. Some cases of rheumatoid arthritis can involve other body parts, including the heart, kidneys, arteries, and lungs. This disease is known for its flare-ups and remissions.

Patient complaints
Your patient may feel poorly, which can lower his or her resistance to the pain. Keep this in mind when you are trying to understand your loved one's discomfort. Some sufferers are unwilling to move their affected body parts. This is dangerous, because movement is necessary to maintain as much joint action as possible. Your patient may complain of heat, redness, swelling, and pain in one or more joints. Accurate diagnosis should be made by the physician or rheumatologist.

Treatment
There is no cure, but there are therapies to help bring relief (see osteoarthritis above). Drugs are the mainstay of treatment during flare-ups. Types used include aspirin in high doses, nonsteroidal anti-inflammatory drugs (NSAID), penicillamine, and gold therapy for more serious cases. Sometimes injections are used to treat specific joints. Know that overuse of injections can actually damage a joint—yet can be helpful when used judiciously. Acute cases may need hospitalization.

Care tips. See osteoarthritis.
For more arthritis information, learn as much as you can about this illness and the latest treatments. The following sources can help you.

The Arthritis Foundation
See Chapter 14.

National Institute of Arthritis, Diabetes,
Digestive and Kidney Diseases
Information Office
9000 Rockville Pike
Building 31, Rm. 9A04
Bethesda, Md. 20205
Ask for publication list.

Confusion

Some years ago, when I was in college, I encountered an elderly woman whose image and behavior have stayed with me to this day. We were seated next to each other on a subway train in New York City. When the train reached our stop, we both got out and walked up the staircase to the street. Then, suddenly, the woman moved toward me, gripped my arm, and said, "I don't know where I am. I don't recognize anything. Please help me." She was more than lost; the woman was confused and disoriented. Instinctively, I tried to reorient her to the neighborhood. "This is Fourteenth Street in Manhattan," I said. "We're across from May's department store. Where did you want to go?" She processed my words as her eyes expressed a mixture of fear and embarrassment. I touched her arm gently and waited a few moments. "Oh, yes, I remember now," she said as the color returned to her face. "I came here to go shopping." With that she disappeared into the crowd.

I remember thinking that the woman's confusion and memory lapse were an expected result of aging. "It'll probably happen to me," I thought. If the same notion had crossed your mind, reconsider it. *The fact is that confusion and severe memory loss should not be seen as acceptable or inevitable.*

Recent figures paint an optimistic picture. Of the 26 million Americans presently over sixty-five, only about 10% display even mild to moderate memory loss. Only about 5% show serious intellectual impairment.

Yes, there are some mental changes that can be attributed to getting older, but they are annoyances to which most older adults adjust, annoyances such as occasional memory loss and a slowing down in the ability to retrieve thoughts.

My concern is that the "senility stereotype," what with its memory losses and intellectual decline, may be keeping some older adults from getting the proper medical evaluation and care they need to avert severe mental impairment. For example, confusion, forgetfulness, disorientation, and agitation may be caused by underlying illnesses, medication side effects, or emotional problems. In many cases, the discovery of underlying treatable illnesses can alleviate, often reverse, the troublesome symptoms.

Also, it is important to pinpoint, if possible, the reason for your older relative's mental changes, because there is the possibility that they may be due to *dementia*—that is, a significant drop in your relative's intellectual ability that interferes with daily functioning. You may see dramatic changes in your loved one's judgment, speaking coordination, vocabulary, math ability, and abstract thinking. Some of the diseases that cause these symptoms are treatable. Others are not. However, sometimes complications can be minimized with appropriate supportive measures (giving your loved one the proper cues to reorient to reality and stir memory, structured schedules, etc.).

How will you know when your older relative's mental changes are no longer "normal"? When his or her confusion or intellectual decline go beyond the boundaries of occasional memory loss and slower thought. Watch for difficulties in thinking, learning, or personality changes. Remember that emotional pressures such as stress, depression, or grief can precipitate confused behavior.

One final warning: Don't underestimate the potential effect of any drug on an elderly person's nervous system. All drugs your loved one is taking should be evaluated by a physician to see if they may be contributing to mental difficulties. Combinations of drugs can cause trouble. And so can over-the-counter preparations, such as cough syrups with alcohol.

If you are concerned about an elderly relative, you should know that the reason for the troublesome symptoms can be diagnosed.

Proper evaluation includes a medical and neurological examination, a look at your loved one's living situation, emotional health, current medications, treatments, and remaining abilities. Everyone deserves to be assessed properly to see if there is a treatment for his or her condition. If a medical assessment is not made your relative risks the persistence of a problem that may be treatable if found early enough, and irreversible, if not.

Where should you turn for a proper evaluation? Ask your family physician. He or she may be able to do the evaluation or refer you to a professional who can. Also, try your local hospital and ask for the names of doctors qualified to evaluate people suspected of dementing illnesses. If a call to the main switchboard fails to reveal the proper source, contact the hospital's public relations' office.

Dementing Illnesses

Alzheimer's Disease

This disease causes about half of the known cases of dementia. It is an ailment of undetermined origin. No one knows what starts the Alzheimer's process or how to stop the mental and physical decline that comes with it. This condition may start with an almost imperceptible deterioration of intellectual powers and a gradual downswing of physical health.

At first your relative may have difficulty remembering things. He or she may have trouble learning new skills or making calculations. There may be some personality changes, perhaps depression. Your loved one may show loss of interest for things he or she used to find diverting. You may witness your relative's sudden angry outbursts or extreme forgetfulness.

Early symptoms may go almost unnoticed, but when the illness is advanced your loved one may be severely impaired. He or she may be incontinent, fall often, be unable to walk, barely speak, recognize very few people.

Alzheimer's ends in death in about seven to ten years. Its pace depends on the patient. Let me also add that although this disease affects older adults mostly, it can strike as early as the mid-forties. A complete medical and neurological examination must be made to properly diagnose the condition.

If your relative has been diagnosed as having Alzheimer's disease, learn as much as you can about the illness. The more you know and the more professional advice you receive, the easier it will be to create a humane and efficient care plan.

Some things for you to remember:

• This illness does not only affect the patient; it can deeply distress the care giver and family. Therefore, it is essential that you and other household members receive as much assistance from relatives, friends, and support groups as possible. Support groups especially can provide an opportunity for you to share your frustration and sorrow with others in situations similar to yours. Contact the Alzheimer's Disease and Related Diseases Association for more information, names of groups in your area, and medical professionals qualified to help (see addresses below).

• Confused patients benefit from a structured environment. Create a consistent schedule that has a simple routine for meals, medication, and other activities. Regular routines will help your loved one to learn what to expect.

• Create a calm atmosphere at home. Keep your voice easy-going when talking to your patient. Always tell him or her what you are doing and why. Allow your patient to participate in decisions as much as possible. Never talk about your patient in front of him or her.

• Use touch to reassure your loved one. Embrace, stroke, hold hands—any affectionate gesture. This will enhance your patient's feelings of security and safety.

• Focus on the tasks your patient can perform. His or her skills will not diminish all at once. Encourage your loved one to make the most of remaining skills.

• Remember your loved one's forgetfulness can cause safety hazards. He or she may forget to shut off appliances, water faucets, etc. Stay alert.

• Provide cues to help your loved one tune in to the moment.

Repeat instructions frequently. Keep sentimental objects and family photos around to activate memories.

• Watch for evidence of falls or other accidents. Your patient's condition may make it impossible for him or her to remember an accident. So watch for bruises, burns, and injuries to the head.

• Learn as much as you can about managing your loved one at home. Try these superior sources: The Alzheimer's Disease and Related Diseases Association (ADRDA), 360 N. Michigan, Chicago, Ill. 60601 (in addition to educational materials they can provide you with a list of physicians in your area who can help); *The 36-Hour Day: A Family Guide to Caring for Persons with Alzheimer's*, by Nancy Mare and Peter V. Rabins, M.D., The Johns Hopkins University Press, 1981; *Managing the Person with Intellectual Loss at Home* (write for this booklet to the Burke Rehabilitation Center, 785 Mamaroneck Ave., White Plains, N.Y. 10165).

Other Causes of Confusion and Dementia

It used to be said that hardening of the arteries leads to old-age dementia. Scientists now tell us that this isn't the cause at all. The actual cause is strokes occurring in the brain again and again, ultimately ruining small sections of it.

This type of dementia is categorized as multi-infarct dementia. The physical and emotional effects of this dementia depend on the area of the brain that has been affected. Your loved one may display difficulties with speech, memory, and coordination. Deterioration usually takes place gradually and may be halted with proper diagnosis and the prevention of future strokes. In some cases nothing can be done to lessen the condition's progress.

There are also many *health conditions* that can cause mental changes. Certain ones respond to treatment. Others will not. Your relative will need a complete physical assessment to determine if an underlying health condition is the culprit. Consider these possibilities: kidney problems, brain infections, brain tumors or injury, medication side effects, multiple sclerosis, thyroid conditions.

Depression, too, can create dementialike symptoms. Indeed there are many things that can contribute to an older adult's feelings of depression: personal losses, such as of a spouse, or child, financial difficulties, physical impairments, poor health, loss of independence, fears of burdening relatives and friends with care needs—the list is long. Because it is easy to miss depression as a significant cause of dementia, it is essential that your patient be given a complete physical and emotional evaluation by a highly qualified physician. When depression is pinpointed as the cause it frequently responds to treatment—and the dementialike symptoms can be reversed.

Know, too, that a dementing illness itself, such as Alzheimer's, can leave its sufferer depressed. A physician experienced in these matters should be able to differentiate whether symptoms of depression are the result of a dementing illness or something else entirely.

Fractures

What should you do if your elderly relative has sustained a fall and you suspect a hip fracture? Watch for these signs: pain in the upper thigh, with the leg rolled outward and the outer edge of the foot lying on the ground. Your loved one may be in shock. Watch for pale, clammy skin and rapid, shallow breathing. Treat for shock (see Chapter 10). Elevate the uninjured leg if shock appears severe. Call an ambulance. Immobilize the fractured limb when patient is transported.

What if you are the elderly person and you're alone after a bad fall? Try to reach for a pillow, blanket, even newspapers or magazines to cover yourself and prevent chilling. Call for help. (As suggested above, "beepers" are available to signal help during an emergency.)

Stroke

Stroke, or cerebral vascular accident, is a serious illness that may leave your loved one partially or completely disabled. Let me reassure you that many stroke victims make significant improvement and go on to lead full lives again. Others could make better progress if they and their home-care givers were more informed about the recovery process and the potential for reversal. Only a few stroke patients remain completely incapacitated because of their illness.

Note: Stroke does not strike only older adults. It can hit younger ones as well, although this happens less frequently. On these next pages I will be speaking to relatives of the elderly, yet the advice is appropriate to stroke patients of all ages.

What is a stroke? It happens when there is a sudden interruption of the blood supply to the brain. In the process, some brain cells are damaged. The body functions controlled by these cells are affected. Arteriosclerosis and hypertension can both contribute to this condition.

The stroke may be triggered by a blood clot blocking the flow of blood or a hemorrhage (blood escapes when an arterial wall breaks).

What are the warning signs? Dizziness, one-sided weakness, and unexplained falls often occur before a stroke. The victim may frequently drop objects. Blood pressure may be high before a stroke, too. A ministroke may result in temporary slurred speech, numbness, confusion, and blurred vision. These signs can show that a major stroke is on its way soon.

If your patient suffers paralysis or weakness he or she can be helped to recover many lost abilities through rehabilitation. It's important to know that most stroke patients who are paralyzed on their left or right sides can learn to walk again and can relearn daily activities.

Rehabilitation after a stroke is hard work. Progress takes time and achievements may be small at first. Some disabilities disappear; others may be permanent. Know some of the things to expect during your patient's convalescence at home so that you can supply intelligent and reassuring support.

Your loved one may behave differently after his or her stroke because the brain handles thinking and feeling. Some possible reactions include involuntary laughing or crying, depression, temper tantrums, irritability, and loss of interest in favorite pastimes.

If your loved one seems excessively irritable, ask the physician how well your patient can be expected to control his or her feelings. There are times when a temper can boil over and out of control. Much has to do with frustrations that can come when your patient has a tough time doing things that were done effortlessly before the stroke. Tip: Take the time to show your loved one easier ways to perform activities to lessen his or her sense of defeat. What if your patient has an inappropriate outburst? Kindly but assertively ask him or her to stop. Express warmth and compassion at these times.

Crying uncontrollably may come from constant feelings of defeat or depressing thoughts. Don't reproach your loved one. Just ask him or her to stop. Your tender commands may help your patient regain control.

Laughing, too, may appear at inappropriate times. Know that your loved one may be very embarrassed by it. Reassure him or her that stroke patients often have this problem.

In the event of paralysis or weakness, rehabilitation will be needed to help your patient regain as much lost ability as possible. Turn to nurses (physician's referral, visiting nurse service, etc.), physical therapists, or occupational therapists for help. Again, the physician may be able to refer you to an experienced and highly qualified individual. Also, to verify the credentials of a therapist, or simply to locate one in your area who can help you, write to the American Physical Therapy Association, 1156 15th St. N.W., Suite 500, Washington, D.C. 20005 or the American Occupational Therapy Association, 1383 Piccard Dr., Rockville, Md. 20850.

To learn more about stroke and how to best help your patient, contact your local heart association for education materials (see phone directory for local listing) or write to the national headquarters at American Heart Association, 7320 Greenville Ave., Dallas, Tex. 75231.

In addition, you may want to check out *Care of the Patient with a Stroke: Handbook for the Patient's Family and the Nurse*, by Genevieve W. Smith, Springer, New York, 1976, or *Stroke: The New Help and the New Life*, by Arthur S. Freese, Random House, New York, 1980.

Parkinson's Disease

Parkinson's disease is a slow chronic condition that affects the nervous system. Its cause is unknown and there is no cure. There are, however, drugs that can help control some of its upsetting symptoms.

What are the signs? At the start of the illness you may notice that your older relative is moving slower than usual. Later, tremors, shuffling gait, and a masklike appearance of the face will develop. Once the disease progresses, muscle rigidity and tremors increase. Your loved one may have difficulty standing, walking, or starting to walk. In time the tongue may be affected by tremors. Speech may be altered and your patient may drool.

The longer the disease continues the more likely your patient will be dependent on others for help. However, it is essential to help your patient maintain as much independence as possible.

Care tips

Learn as much as you can about this illness. Check out *Parkinson's Disease: A Guide for Patient and Family*, by Robert C. Duvoisin, Raven Press, New York, 1978. Also write the National Institute of Neurological and Communicative Disorders and Strokes (see Chapter 14) and the American Parkinson Disease Association, 116 John St., New York, N.Y. 10038 for publications.

The occupational therapist can help your patient manage personal care tasks and other aspects of daily living. You must encourage your loved one and help him or her with exercises prescribed by professionals. There may be times when watching your loved one having difficulty with a simple task will be heartbreaking for you. Although your instinct may be to run over and help, resist it. Your constant interference may make your relative feel exceedingly dependent, and this can cause him or her emotional difficulties. Give as much love and understanding as you can. Your relative will need this as the illness progresses.

Know that stress and anxiety can aggravate the symptoms of your patient's illness. Try to create a calm and accepting atmosphere at home.

Know that the muscular activity caused by tremors may lessen your patient's tolerance to heat. Adjust the thermostat to a comfortable temperature. Make sure your loved one is not overdressed.

Know that as Parkinson's disease progresses, drooling and chewing may be a problem. Encourage your patient to feed himself or herself as long as possible.

Know that many Parkinson's patients have to urinate frequently. Be sure that your elderly relative's room is close to a bathroom. Constipation can also be a problem for these patients, so be alert to it. Lack of activity and certain medications can contribute to the condition. Ask the physician how to manage the problem.

Know that despite your loved one's masklike expression and other disturbing symptoms of the disease, Parkinson's does not affect intelligence. It may be difficult for your patient to participate in activities he or she may find distracting. In time, boredom may increase, so you will need to find ways to offer your patient intelligent stimulation. Consult the physician.

There are drugs available that may ease some of your patient's disturbing symptoms. Unfortunately, with the potential for offering relief, these drugs can also bring a host of discomforting and sometimes dangerous side effects. Therefore it is essential that patients on anti-Parkinson's medications be carefully and continually monitored by their physicians. For more information about the side effects of the drugs prescribed for your loved one refer to the *Physician's Desk Reference* and/or the *United States Pharmacopeia/Dispensing Information* as discussed in Chapter 3.

Here's a rundown of the most common anti-Parkinson's medications and how they may affect your patient.

Carbi-dopa is increasingly becoming the treatment of choice for many Parkinson's patients. It is a combination of an anticholinergic and dopamine. This union enhances the activity of the dopamine, thereby requiring lower doses of the medication and resulting in fewer side effects than the other traditionally used anti-Parkinson's medications (see below). Sinemet is the usual trademark name. The most common side effect in the early stages of treatment is confusion. The drug is administered in small doses to start and should be carefully and continually monitored by the physician.

Levadopa (L-dopa) has been successful in easing many of the symptoms of Parkinson's, but its side effects can interfere with treatment. These include nausea, involuntary movements, and postural hypotension. Add to that the fact that foods high in vitamin B-6 can reduce the effectiveness of L-dopa. That means patients on this drug must be told to avoid foods such as prunes, powdered skim milk, sweet potatoes, tuna fish, pork, bacon, oatmeal, liver, and dried fruits. Carbi-dopa can be taken with vitamin B-6 without adverse reactions, however.

Anticholinergics comprise another group of drugs that may control some Parkinson's symptoms. Again, however, the side effects interfere with successful treatment. Artane, Cogentin, and Disipal fall into this group. Their side effects include confusion, hallucinations and other mental changes, and urinary retention. These drugs should not be given to patients with certain kinds of heart disease or glaucoma. Also, sudden withdrawal from these medications can be dangerous.

Do you need more information on the subject of older adults? Call your nearest United Way office (check phone listings). They have a directory of the United Way information and referral services across the United States. The information and referral service can put you in touch with programs and services for older adults in your part of the country. Ask the telephone information operator for the phone number of the Federal Information Center. If there isn't a listing in your town, try the nearest large city. The center can provide you with information regarding agencies, programs, and publications of the United States government. Also, any of the following organizations may prove helpful.

ACTION
806 Connecticut Ave.
Washington, D.C. 20525

This group administers a foster grandparent program.

Administration on Aging
Office of Human Development Services
330 Independence Ave., S.W.
Washington, D.C. 20201

American Association of Retired Persons
1909 K Street N.W.
Washington, D.C. 20049

Asociación Nacional Pro Personas Mayores
1730 W. Olympic Blvd.
Los Angeles, Calif. 90015

This is the national association for the Hispanic elderly.

Gray Panthers
3635 Chestnut St.
Philadelphia, Pa. 19104

This is an organization of young, middle-aged, and elderly activists which tries to solve problems of older adults through action and social change.

National Association of Area Agencies on Aging
600 Maryland Ave., S.W.
Suite 208
Washington, D.C. 20024

National Center on Black Aging
1424 K Street, N.W.
Washington, D.C. 20005

National Council of Senior Citizens
925-15th St., N.W.
Washington, D.C. 20005

This is a coalition of 4,000 activist groups that work for government legislation to help the elderly and also administers numerous programs for the low-income elderly.

National Pacific/Asian Resource Center on Aging
811 First Ave.
Coleman Bldg.
Seattle, Wash. 98104

This is an advocacy group that focuses on improving social and health services for older adults who are Pacific/Asian.

13

Caring for a Loved One Who Has a Terminal Illness

For many people, life ends in the loneliness of an alien and sterile hospital room. Medical care may be good, but there is often an inadequate amount of emotional warmth and human contact. Fortunately, home care can provide an alternative to this. So, too, can hospice care, a care concept that focuses on the quality, not the length, of the patient's remaining life. In fact, thanks to a provision of the omnibus tax reform bill, President Reagan has signed legislation to make hospice care an eligible expense under Medicare. More good news is that many private insurance companies, including Blue Cross/Blue Shield, are developing and enacting reimbursement programs that may ultimately cover a significant amount of hospice-care costs.

Home care for a dying patient may seem frightening and overwhelming. Your relative's fears and anxieties about death may be as debilitating as the illness itself. Moreover, in addition to suffering from pain, loneliness, dependency, and loss of control, your relative may feel guilty about burdening you with the tasks of care.

You may wonder how to cope with your grief and provide care at the same time. How should you act when you are with your loved one? What should you tell the children? How will you manage when your loved one is gone?

Without a doubt caring for a relative who is terminally ill can be very traumatic. You may need the support of your clergyman or perhaps a professional therapist. You will certainly need the understanding of your family and friends.

This chapter is designed to help improve your coping skills at this time and to better your understanding of your loved one's feelings.

This is, of course, an extremely sensitive and painful subject. You may be able to work through your grief by reading books by authorities in the field. I, personally, have found the books of Elisabeth Kübler-Ross comforting and inspiring. Kübler-Ross practiced general medicine in Switzerland before coming to the United States. Her work with the dying and her books about her experiences may illuminate your understanding of death and enable you to communicate more effectively with your terminally ill patient. Consider reading *On Death and Dying*, New York: Macmillan, 1969, and *Questions and Answers on Death and Dying*, New York: Macmillan, 1974. Other books you may find of interest are *The Experience of Dying* by E. Mansell Pattison, New Jersey: Prentice-Hall, 1977; *Home Care: Living with Dying*, by Elizabeth R. Pritchard, New York: Columbia University Press, 1980; and *When Bad Things Happen to Good People*, by Harold S. Kushner, New York: Schocken, 1982.

How Can You Best Support Your Loved One?

Let me begin with the most important thing: the diagnosis. If your loved one is told that he or she has a disease that will inevitably lead to death, be sure to get at least one second opinion. We have all heard stories of a "terminally ill" patient who was *mis*diagnosed.

Once the illness is confirmed to your satisfaction, your next question may be, "How long does my loved one have to live?" Know that no matter how qualified and experienced the physician, he or she cannot accurately predict the time of your loved one's death.

A nurse who attends to the needs of many dying patients told me the story of a fifty-five-year-old gentleman whose doctor had given him two months to live. The gentleman, understandably hopeless, mustered his courage to put his papers in order, draw up a will, and say good-bye to friends and family. *That was a year ago.* He continues living to this day and maintaining hope.

Said the nurse: "Who owns God's calendar?" Good question. No one does. Not the doctors or the nurses or the family.

Learn as much as you can about your loved one's condition so that you are aware of the available treatments. Contact organizations that provide patient education materials about your loved one's illness (the American Cancer Society, the American Heart Association, etc.). Speak to highly qualified medical specialists. Let me suggest that, if possible, you do not make a final decision about treatment the day your relative receives the diagnosis. The reason: This is the moment when care givers and their patients undergo the most shock. It is anything but a time of clear-headedness and objectivity. Wait a brief while until you are more calm.

Once you have determined which treatments, if any, will be administered, be sure that you and your patient understand their effects. What will the quality of your loved one's life be after the treatment? Will you need special instructions in after-care? Does your loved one fully understand its repercussions? Do you?

Next, of course, is the actual care of your loved one at home. You will need to know how to manage his or her medical needs. The physician should be able to give you explicit instructions. Carrying out specific tasks may not be easy. You may be asked to administer mouth care, bladder and bowel care, ostomy care— any one of a number of things depending on your patient's condition. Visiting nurses and other skilled care givers can be especially helpful at this time.

Additionally, some hospitals have home-care training programs where care givers are taught how to manage their terminally ill relatives. Investigate the hospitals in your area for the programs they may offer.

What about your loved one's emotional needs? There can be no simple advice here. Every patient is unique and needs a highly individualized brand of loving care at this time. There are, however, some things for you to consider. For example, I've heard relatives of terminally ill patients say, "Maybe I should quit my job and stop all other activities to stay home with my husband/ wife/etc. full time." Indeed, some patients may expect their families to "drop everything" and provide round-the-clock care and companionship. I believe, and the many authorities to whom I have spoken concur, that you should try to continue your own normal pattern of life as long as possible. Yes, you may have to alter your schedule somewhat if you are the primary care giver, but you risk emotional and physical hazards if you insist on putting yourself on twenty-four-hour duty. Your time away from the home will help you maintain your own internal support system. Clearly, you will need other activities in order to re-energize and sustain quality care.

Good communication between you and your patient is also very important at this time. Your loved one is probably over- flowing with feelings. Encourage him or her to express them. The process of ventilating emotion may enable your relative to gradually come to terms with his or her illness and death. This communication doesn't just help the patient—it can help you, too. Seeing your loved one face dying with dignity and strength may enhance your own courage. As one young man said about his father, "Dad's been remarkable. How can I do any less?"

Of course, communicativeness does not come easily to every- one, so don't push your relative into conversation unless he or she is interested. You can, however, try to induce conversation by creating an atmosphere of acceptance and reassurance. Be attentive to your loved one's words. Establish closeness by hold- ing his or her hand. Be demonstrative.

You can also help by activating the spirit of hope in your patient and family. Even when illness is unstoppable, hopeless- ness should not be allowed to weave its way into your lives.

There may be surgery or treatments that can be tried. There is the hope that additional treatments will work, that a cure will be found. There is the kind of hope that enables a patient to survive until an important event arrives, such as a wedding or the birth of a child; or the hope that there will be time to say all the things the patient wants to say to cherished family members and friends. Hope can be magic. It can remove the agony from terminal illness.

It is also important that you get in touch with your own feelings about dying and death. If you are having trouble dealing with your feelings you may be relaying this attitude to your patient. He or she may pick up your anxieties and fears. This can burden your relative and make it more difficult for him or her to cope. There are clues to let you know you are in trouble—elevated levels of anxiety, depression, sleeping difficulties, job problems, physical illness, and bouts of weeping. These signs are hardly unusual during a traumatic time, but their *persistence* may be hazardous to your emotional and physical health—and your loved one.

What Is Your Loved One's World Like at This Time?

This, of course, depends on your relative's coping skills and the nature of his or her illness.

It is natural for anyone diagnosed with a serious illness to experience shock and anxiety at first. Kübler-Ross believes that the dying pass through five stages on their way to death: denial and isolation, anger, depression, and acceptance. Her book *On Death and Dying* explores this theory in much detail. Read it to gain a clearer understanding of your patient—and yourself. Let me add that not all professionals who care for the dying believe that there are five stages. However, this book provides a sensitive and intelligent look at the experiences of the terminally ill.

Another natural reaction is fear of pain and suffering. Terminal illness does not automatically mean severe pain. In fact, many dying patients experience no pain at all. The amount of discomfort will depend on your patient's illness and state of mind. State of mind? Yes, anxiety and depression can lower a person's tolerance for pain. It's crucial that your loved one receives quality pain management and emotional support.

Loss of control, too, may be another concern for your relative. He or she may fear loss of certain body functions, loss of independence. Or perhaps your loved one is so distressed there is a fear of losing his or her mind. Your reassurances will be very much needed. Your patient may also benefit by talking to a clergyman or professional counselor.

Remember, too, that your relative may be concerned about the meaning of death. If he or she does not have strong religious beliefs or notions about an afterlife, the question of what happens after death may be tormenting. In such circumstances, as with any emotional concerns that are burdensome, your relative may require professional help. Again, consider the appropriate clergyman or therapist.

The Hospice Alternative

Hospice is an excellent and humane alternative to the conventional ways of treating the terminally ill. Its name goes back to medieval times when it meant a way station for pilgrims and travelers. It was a place to stop, recoup and be cared for. Today, it is a method of caring for seriously ill people who are going through life's last journey.

The hospice movement was started by Dr. Cicely Saunders of the St. Christopher's Hospice in London, England. Her idea was to care for dying patients in their own homes as long as possible, with back-up in-patient beds available in a comfortable and home-like setting.

Hospice embraces the patient rather than the illness. It tries to enable the terminally ill to live their last moments, weeks, or days as richly as possible. It recognizes the effect terminal illness has on the whole family and attempts to make it less emotionally traumatic for all involved.

Furthermore, hospice goes beyond the methods used in traditional scientific medicine. Its philosophy is that patients should be as comfortable as possible in their last days. Clearly, pain control and easing distressing symptoms are a major part of hospice care. For example, in the hospital, painkilling drugs are usually administered only when a patient requires them. However, the physician supervising hospice care will prescribe painkillers not just to ease pain, but to prevent it. Medication is given on a consistent basis before the pain can reemerge. Of course, there are other physical discomforts associated with terminal illness that need medical attention: loss of appetite, nausea, breathing problems, and many others are attended to as they occur.

Generally speaking, there are three styles of hospice. There's the free-standing type, which is an institution by itself; the in-hospital hospice, which is a hospice located within a hospital setting; and the home-care hospice, where the hospice team visits the patient in his or her own home and administers care there as long as possible, in addition to helping the family with care tasks and with working through grief.

The hospice team? Indeed, there are many professionals who make hospice possible. Hospice care is supervised by a physician and directed by a nurse. Other staff members include medical social workers, physical therapists, occupational therapists, clergymen, and volunteers. Counselors may also be available to provide guidance in areas such as religious matters, financial and legal concerns, estate planning, and funeral counseling. Other services may include homemaking (meal preparation and child care), transportation for shopping, doctor's appointments, other trips, and bereavement follow-up to a family that needs help accepting their loss.

In-patient facilities in a hospital or free-standing institution may be available to provide a back-up location for patients who need more sophisticated medical treatment and supervision that can be offered in the home setting. Sometimes the family can no longer manage their loved one's condition and must transfer the patient to the hospice facility. This may be for only a short time; in many such cases the patient returns home.

To be accepted into a hospice program your loved one will almost always need a statement from his or her physician that says death is expected within six months. As mentioned earlier in this chapter, doctors cannot always tell when a patient will die. To be sure, there are patients who continue on past their physician's original prediction. And there are patients whose illness goes into remission. Hospice patients are usually in the hands of a physician who can determine whether or not additional treatments or therapies are needed.

Two final points to remember: Some physicians are not pro hospice. In certain situations a physician may doubt the quality of an available facility or perhaps be unwilling to give up the care of his or her patient to another service. Learn as much as you can about hospice care and the ones nearest you so that you and your patient can make an informed decision.

Not every terminally ill patient should be expected to be pro hospice. Some people are unwilling to stop therapeutic treatment and commit themselves to the hospice program. Cost, too is a consideration. You are best advised to check your loved one's financial resources and insurance coverage to see if it is feasible to support your patient in the home setting.

Want more information about hospice? Write the National Hospice Organization, 1311A Dolley Madison Blvd., McLean, Va. 22101. This organization provides hospice information and a nationwide listing of hospice programs. You may also find the hospice program in your community by calling visiting nurse associations, local hospitals, and health departments.

When Your Loved One Dies at Home

No matter how much emotional preparation and professional guidance you have had, the death of a loved one at home may fill you and your family with much trauma and confusion.

Therefore, you will want to make certain arrangements ahead

of time. Certainly, this is a very sensitive situation. You may need the help of a trusted friend or relative to make the appropriate decisions.

Your loved one's body will, of course, remain in your home until it is moved elsewhere. This, too, may be exceedingly stressful for you. There are no rules in this situation. Do what comes most naturally to you. You may wish to stay near the body, hold it, cover it. You may prefer to leave the room until assistance arrives. Whatever works for you is best.

Ask the physician who should be called at the time of your loved one's death. You may be told to call the county coroner, sheriff or physician, depending on the law in your area, to make an official pronouncement of death. Once an official visits your home to make the pronouncement, your loved one's body will be transported to the mortuary or funeral home.

Bereavement

Death is a reality we all must accept. Your loved one's death may fill you with sorrow. You may feel relieved that his or her ordeal is over. You may miss your loved one very much and yet feel peace within yourself. As always, there are many possibilities. You are unique and so are your feelings.

Death, of course, can feel like a terrible tragedy, and your grief may interfere with your ability to function properly. Bereavement counseling may be necessary to help you work through your feelings and accept your loss. A therapist, social worker, or clergyman may be able to help you or perhaps refer you to a suitable professional. Indeed, there are sensitively trained professionals who can offer counseling based on their expert knowledge of the grieving and recovery process. Don't hesitate to reach out for help.

14

Additional Resources

More than fifty information sources are listed below. They will put you in touch with health-related organizations that can give you the information and support you need to manage a loved one's health-care needs at home. These sources, of course, are in addition to the ones already offered in the preceding chapters.

Alcoholics Anonymous
c/o AA World Service, Inc.
P.O. Box 459
Grand Central Station
New York, N.Y. 10163

The American Association for Marriage and Family Therapy
1717 K St. N.W.
Washington, D.C. 20006

This organization will give you referrals to qualified therapists.

American Cancer Society
777 Third Ave.
New York, N.Y. 10017

Association for the Severely Handicapped
7010 Roosevelt Way N.E.
Seattle, Wash. 98115

This association provides information about educational opportunities for severely handicapped individuals.

American Association of Homes for the Aging
1050 17th St. N.W.
Suite 770
Washington, D.C. 20036

Write for information about nonprofit, community-sponsored housing, homes for the aging, and health-related facilities serving the elderly.

American Diabetic Association
2 Park Ave.
New York, N.Y. 10016

Write for patient education materials.

American Digestive Disease Society
7720 Wisconsin Ave.
Bethesda, Md. 20814

This organization provides information about specific functional disorders, diagnosis, and treatment; it sponsors GUTLINE, a call-in counseling service, available Tuesday and Thursday evenings from 7:30 P.M. to 9:00 P.M., where a physician offers advice.

American Heart Association
7320 Greenville Ave.
Dallas, Tex. 75231

The national chapter provides patient education materials.

American Liver Foundation
998 Pompton Ave.
Cedar Grove, N.J. 07009

Write for patient education materials about pediatric and adult liver disorders; referrals to support groups.

American Lung Association
1740 Broadway
New York, N.Y. 10019

Ask for information about lung diseases such as emphysema, tuberculosis, asthma.

American Lupus Society
23751 Madison St.
Torrance, Calif. 90505

This organization supplies patient education materials.

American Occupational Therapy Association, Inc.
1383 Piccard Dr.
Rockville, Md. 20850

Contact to verify credentials of certified therapists.

American Printing House for the Blind, Inc.
1839 Frankfort Ave.
P.O. Box 6085
Louisville, Ky. 40206

This organization supplies educational aids and books for the blind, catalogues for products in Braille, large-type products.

American Psychiatric Association
Publication Sales
1700 18th St. N.W.
Washington, D.C. 20009

Ask for publication list dealing with many areas of mental health including specific illnesses, treatment, and medications.

American Red Cross
18th and D St. N.W.
Washington, D.C. 20006

Write for publication list for home-care and related books.

Amyotrophic Lateral Sclerosis Society of America
15300 Ventura Blvd.
Sherman Oaks, Calif. 91403

Ask for patient education materials.

Arthritis Foundation
1314 Spring St. N.W.
Atlanta, Ga. 30309

Association for Brain Tumor Research
6232 N. Pulaski Rd.
Suite 200
Chicago, Ill. 60646

This organization supplies brochures about various types of brain tumor and their treatment.

Asthma and Allergy Foundation of America
9604 Wisconsin Ave.
Suite 100
Bethesda, Md. 20814

This group offers pamphlets about asthma and specific food and drug allergies, and oversees eighteen different chapters across the country for community programs.

Association for the Education of the Visually Handicapped
206 N. Washington St.
Alexandria, Va. 22314

Contact for referrals to organizations and professionals who
specialize in education of the visually handicapped.

Braille Institute of America
741 N. Vermont Ave.
Los Angeles, Calif. 90029

Cancer Counseling and Research Center
6060 N. Central Expressway
Suite 140
Dallas, Tex. 75206

Ask for information about their unique program that teaches
cancer patients and their families to better manage the psychological repercussions of the illness. The center supplies referrals
to professionals throughout the country specially trained to provide therapy.

Candlelighters
2025 Eye St. N.W.
Suite 1011
Washington, D.C. 20006

An organization of parents of children with cancer that provides
information about childhood and teenage cancer, support groups,
etc.

Center for Science in the Public Interest
1755 S St. N.W.
Washington, D.C. 20009

Ask for their publication list on food and nutrition.

Center for Studies of Schizophrenia
National Institute of Mental Health
Parklawn Bldg., Rm. 10-95
5600 Fisher's Lane
Rockville, Md. 20857

Write for the latest research information.

Committee to Combat Huntington's Disease, Inc.
250 West 57th St.
New York, N.Y. 10107

This organization provides patient education materials, support
for families, and referrals to physicians and support groups.

Consumer Information Center
Pueblo, Col. 81009

The center offers a wide variety of health-related publications;
ask for publication list.

Cystic Fibrosis Foundation
6000 Executive Blvd.
Suite 309
Rockville, Md. 20852

The Down Syndrome Congress
1640 West Roosevelt Rd.
Chicago, Ill. 60608

Ask for information about support groups for parents, siblings,
and individuals with Down syndrome, and for publication list.

Dysautonomia Foundation, Inc.
370 Lexington Ave.
New York, N.Y. 10017

This organization supplies treatment manuals for parents, physicians, and nurses. Write for publication list.

Emphysema Anonymous
P.O. Box 66
Ft. Myers, Fla. 33902

This is an organization for anyone with breathing problems. It offers education, encouragement, and mutual support to those with emphysema and related breathing disorders.

Epilepsy Foundation of America
4351 Garden City Dr.
Suite 406
Landover, Md. 20785

Hadley School for the Blind
700 E. Elm St.
Winnetka, Ill. 60093

This organization offers a Braille correspondence course.

International Association of Laryngectomees
c/o American Cancer Society
777 Third Ave.
New York, N.Y. 10017

Leukemia Society of America, Inc.
Public Education and Information
800 Second Ave.
New York, N.Y. 10017

The Living Bank
P.O. Box 6725
Houston, Tex. 77265

This organization helps individuals donate organs and tissues to people in need.

Mental Health Association
National Headquarters
1800 N. Kent St.
Arlington, Va. 22209

Ask for their pamphlet *Helping the Mental Patient at Home.*

Multiple Sclerosis Society National Headquarters
205 East 42nd St.
New York, N.Y. 10017

Muscular Dystrophy Association
810 Seventh Ave.
New York, N.Y. 10019

Myasthenia Gravis Foundation, Inc.
15 East 26th St.
New York, N.Y. 10010

National Association of the Deaf
814 Thayer Ave.
Silver Spring, Md. 20910

Contact for pamphlets on devices to aid the deaf, communication with a deaf person, and other educational materials.

National Association for Sickle Cell Disease
3460 Wilshire Blvd.
Suite 1012
Los Angeles, Calif. 90010

National Association of Patients
    on Hemodialysis and Transplantation, Inc.
156 William St.
New York, N.Y. 10038

This organization supplies information about renal failure, current treatments, available resources, and individual chapters.

National Cancer Information Service Hotline
Toll-free telephone number: 1-800-638-6694

This service will refer callers to local cancer organizations.

National Cancer Institute
Office of Cancer Communications
Bldg. 31, Rm. 10A18
Bethesda, Md. 20205

Publication lists on cancer, diagnosis, and treatment are available here.

National Homecaring Council, Inc.
235 Park Ave. So.
New York, N.Y. 10003

Write for publication list on homemaker and home health-aide services.

National Foundation for Ileitis and Colitis, Inc.
295 Madison Ave.
New York, N.Y. 10017

National Hemophilia Foundation
19 West 34th St.
Rm. 1204
New York, N.Y. 10001

National Institute for Burn Medicine
909 East Ann
Ann Arbor, Mich. 48104

This organization provides education materials about burn care for laypersons and professionals.

National Institutes of Health
9000 Rockville Pike
Bethesda, Md. 20205

Address your letter to the Public Information Office of the institute that deals with the topic that interests you: National Institute on Aging; National Institute of Allergy and Infectious Diseases; National Institute of Arthritis, Diabetes, Digestive and Kidney Diseases; National Cancer Institute; National Institute of Child Health; National Institute of Dental Research; National Eye Institute; National Heart, Lung and Blood Institute; National Institute of Neurological and Communicative Disorders and Strokes.

National Kidney Foundation
2 Park Ave.
New York, N.Y. 10016

National Reye's Syndrome Foundation
P.O. Box 829
Bryan, Ohio 43506

The National Retinitis Pigmentosa Foundation
  Fighting Blindness
8331 Mindale Circle
Baltimore, Md. 21207

National Self-Help Clearinghouse
Graduate School and University Center
  of the City University of New York
33 West 42nd St.
Rm. 1227
New York, N.Y. 10036

This organization provides information or referrals to those in need of the supportive assistance of self-help groups; write to the above address or phone 212-840-7606.

National Spinal Cord Injury Association
369 Elliot St.
Newton Upper Falls, Mass. 02164

Ask for patient education brochures, especially the *Handbook for Paraplegic and Quadriplegic Individuals*.

Recordings for the Blind, Inc.
215 East 58th St.
New York, N.Y. 10022

This organization offers more than 58,000 recorded textbooks for visually handicapped students at all grade levels; ask for the list pertaining to the subject and grade level you need.

Ronald McDonald Houses
National Coordinator
500 N. Michigan Ave.
Chicago, Ill. 60611

Write for more information about these homes away from home for parents and families of children being treated for serious illnesses at nearby hospitals. There are more than forty such houses around the country.

The Self-Help Center
1600 Dodge Ave.
Suite S-122
Evanston, Ill. 60201

Offers self-help publications and referrals to individuals seeking self-help groups and wanting to start new ones.

United Cerebral Palsy Association, Inc.
66 East 34th St.
New York, N.Y. 10016

This organization supplies a wide variety of information for individuals of all ages with cerebral palsy, including patient education materials, career development, and housing advice.

Index

Abdominal rigidness, 118
Active exercises, 42
Activity, 96
    post-surgical, 150–151, 156
Adenoidectomy, 165
Administering medication, 60–68
Adolescents, chronically-ill, 194–195. *See also* Child care
Adult day care programs, 31, 286–287
Aging, 276–277. *See also* Elderly patients
Alcohol, 131
    and drug interaction, 68
Alcoholics Anonymous, 274
Alcoholism, 250, 274
Allergic reactions, 123–124
Alzheimer's disease, 250, 298–300
Ambulances, 229–231
American Cancer Society, 64, 217
American Psychiatric Association, 274
Amputation, 150, 153–154
Amputee wheelchair, 71
Anaphylactic shock, 124, 246–247
Anatomy of an Illness as Perceived by the Patient: Reflections on Healing and Regeneration (Cousins), 28
Angina, 70, 155, 244
Antacids, 68
Antianxiety drugs, 272
Antibiotics, 168
Anticoagulants, 68, 160
Antidepressant medication, 266, 273
Antiemetic drugs, 66, 133

Antipsychotics, 272
Anxiety, 263–264
Apical pulse, 89
Appendectomy, 154
Appetite loss:
    child, 179–180, 198, 199
    elderly, 292–293
    prevention of, 130–133
    radiation and chemotherapy-induced, 64, 65, 130, 133
Arterial surgery, 154
Arthritis, 293–296
    and sex, 211–212
Artificial insemination, 66
Artificial respiration, 228, 235–238
Aspirin, 68, 81, 82, 160
    for children, 62, 167–168, 173
Atherosclerosis, 69, 155
Atrial fibrillation, 89
Autonomic hyperreflexia, 223
Axillary temperature, 86

Bacterial endocarditis, 160–161
Barbiturates, 272
Basic food groups, 126–129
Bathing, 48–53
Bed, 17–18
    adjustment, 20–21
    linens and rails, 21
    and patient movement, 40, 42, 44–46
Bed bath, 49–51
Bedpans, 55–56

331

Bedside commodes, 56–57
Bedsores, 17–18, 39–42, 112
Belching, 105–106
Bladder control, loss of, 57–58, 121–122
Bleeding, 101, 121
    discharge, 101
    emergency, 234–235
    internal, 234–235
Blender cooking, 135–136
Blood clotting, and chemotherapy, 65
Blood pressure reading, 90–94
Blue Cross/Blue Shield, 309
Body movement, 96–98
Body odor, 114
Body positions, 97–98
Body sounds, 120
Body vibrations, 119
Boredom, 76–79
Bowel control, loss of, 57–58, 122
Brachial pulse, 87–88
Bread/cereal food group, 128, 132, 142
Breakfast, 130
Breast examinations, 226
Breathing changes, 98–100
Breath odor, 114–115
By-pass surgery, 154–156

Cabin fever, 76–79
Caffeine, 36
Calcium, 128
Cancer, 158, 162, 217
    chemotherapy for, 65–66, 140
    mental problems due to, 250
    radiation therapy for, 63–64, 140
Capsules, medicine, 61
Carbi-dopa, 306
Cardiac arrest, 235, 244
Cardio-Pulmonary Resuscitation, 228, 233
    235–238
Care-giving hints, 25–30
Care programs, 31–32, 286–287
Carnation Instant Breakfast, 146
Carotid pulse, 88, 238
Cast care, 48, 53–55
Cataract surgery, 157–158
Catheter care, 58–59
Chemotherapy, 63, 65, 134, 135
    child, 187–188
    diet, 139–140
Cheyne-Stokes respiration, 100

Chicken pox, 166, 167–168, 188
Child care, 166–201
    administering medication, 62, 167–168,
        173, 176, 177, 196–197
    choking, 239
    chronical illnesses, 187–201
    common illnesses, 167–168
    and education, 200–201
    effects on marriage, 197–198
    emotional needs of child, 181–186, 188–
        201
    feeding, 178–180
    fevers, 81, 82, 84, 85, 103, 104, 167, 168,
        171–173
    hospital, 183–186
Child psychologists, 195
Chills, 101–102
Choking victims, 63, 123
    Heimlich Maneuver for, 123, 228, 232,
        239–242
Chronic illness, 187–201
Circulation, cast, 55
City ambulances, 231
Cleaning sickroom, 33–34
Clothing, 34–35
Clues, health, 95–125
Colds, 166, 168–169
Cold therapies, 38–39
Colon resection, 158
Colostomy, 163, 164
    and sex, 218, 220
Coma, diabetic, 242–243
Comatose signs, 107
Comfortably Yours, 76
Commodes, 56–57
Companions, 78–79
Complaints, patient, 121–125
Confusion, elderly, 296–301
Congregate housing, 275, 282, 289–290
Constipation, 59, 105, 142
Convulsions:
    emergency treatment for, 245
    febrile, 171–172
Cooperative care programs, 32
Coronary by-pass patients, 89
Costs:
    emergency room, 233
    home care, 2–3, 21–25
    hospital, 2, 3
    nursing home, 282

Coughing, 99, 153
Cousins, Norman, 28
Cranberry juice, 220
Craniotomy, 158–159
Crutches, 74

Day-care programs, adult, 31, 286–287
Day hospital programs, 286–287
Decubitus ulcers. *See* Bedsores
Dehydration, 111, 169–170
Delusions, 264–265, 269
Dementia, 296–301
Depression, 250, 265–266, 268
 chronically ill child, 198–200
 elderly, 301
 post-surgical, 156
 and sex, 205, 212, 221–222
Diabetic(s):
 bathing feet of, 50–51
 breath odor of, 114, 115
 diet, 140–142
 emergencies, 242–243
 and sex, 212–213
 urine odor of, 116
Diagnostic tests, 186, 224
Diapering, 58
Diarrhea, 64, 105, 144
 child, 169–170
Diet(s), 126–147
 appetite loss, 130–133
 basic food groups, 126–129
 breakfast, 130
 fad, 129
 feeding special patients, 143–144
 and nausea, 133
 nursing home, 281
 recipes, 144–147
 restricted, 136–143
 taste changes, 135
Dieticians, registered, 9, 14–15, 136
Dignity, 27, 58
Dilation and curettage (D & C), 159
Discharge(s), 101
 cast, 54
 odor, 115
Discharge planning, hospital, 7
Disorientation, 106–107
Diuretics, 68
Drugs. *See* Medication
Dry bed bath, 49

Dry climax, 221
Dryness, mouth, 102, 134
Dry skin, 48, 49
Dying patient, 309–317

Ear abnormalities, 103, 124–125
Earaches, 170–171
Edmund Scientific for Health and Fitness, 75
Education of sick child, 200–201
Ejaculation, 194
 problems, 212, 218, 221
Elderly patient(s), 275–308
 aging signs, 276–277
 appetite loss, 292–293
 arthritis, 293–296
 day care, 286–287
 dementia, 277, 296–301
 emotional changes, 277, 296–307
 food services, 287–288
 foster homes, 288
 fractures, 301–302
 home care strategy, 282–291
 living area adapted to, 291–292
 medication, 297, 306–307
 movement of, 47
 nursing homes, 275, 278–282
 Parkinson's disease, 208, 250, 304–307
 professional help for, 283, 286–291, 303–
  304, 305
 special housing arrangements, 289–290
 stereotypes, 276
 transportation and escort services, 290–291
Electric wheelchair, 72
Emergencies:
 ambulances for, 229–231
 bleeding, 234–235
 cardio-pulmonary resuscitation, 228, 233,
  235–238
 defined, 229
 diabetic, 242–243
 emergency room, 232–233
 fainting, 243
 heart attack, 228, 230, 235–238, 242–243
 Heimlich Maneuver, 123, 228, 232, 239–
  242
 instruction, 233
 seizures, 245
 shock, 246–247
 treatment, 227–248
 unconsciousness, 247

while alone, 231–232, 242
Emotions, care-giver, 16, 25–26, 28, 69
  and child care, 189–201
  and elderly patient, 284–286, 303
  and mentally ill, 249, 259–263
  self-help groups for, 8–9, 195
  and terminally ill, 309–317
Emotions, patient, 106–107
  child, 181–186, 188–201
  elderly, 277, 296–307
  post-surgical, 156, 162–164
  and sex, 203, 205–225
  terminally ill, 312–314
Enemas, 59–60
Enterostomal therapist, 163
Entertainment, 76–79
Epinephrine, 247
Equipment, self-help, 74–76
Escort services, 290–291
Exercise, 37–38
Extramarital sex, 215–216
Eye abnormalities, 103, 157–158

Facial movements, 97
Facial surgery, 213
Fad diets, 129
Fainting, 243
Family of elderly patient, 284–286
Family planning, 226
Family support groups, for relatives of
    mentally ill, 257, 258–260, 261
Fashionable, 76
Fatigue:
  care-giver, 16
  post-surgical, 149, 155
Fat-restricted diets, 139
Febrile convulsions, 171–172
Femoral pulse, 88
Fertility, and chemotherapy, 66
Fever, 80–87, 103–104
  child, 81, 82, 84, 85, 103, 104, 167, 168,
    171–173
Fiber intake, 142
Flatulence, 105–106
Flowers in sickroom, 34
Flu, 166
Flushing, 108
Food exchanges, 141–142
Food services, 287–288
Fortified milk, 145

Foster families for mentally ill, 257, 258
Foster homes for elderly, 288
Fracture bedpans, 56
Fractures, elderly, 301–302
Fred Sammons, Inc., 75
Free-standing hospice, 315
Fruit, 127–128, 142
  shake, 146
Funeral homes, 317
Furnishings, sickroom, 18, 20

Gall bladder surgery, 159
Gastrectomy, 160
Gay organizations, 225
German measles, 173–174
Gown, 34
Group Health Association of America, 23
Guilt, care-giver, 26–27, 69, 189, 284–285
Gynecologists, 208, 226

Hair loss:
  and chemotherapy, 65–66
  post-surgical, 149
Hallucinations, 106, 269–271
Health, importance of, 9
Health clues, 95–125
Health insurance, 21–25, 309. *See also
    specific plans*
Health Insurance Association of America, 22
Health maintenance organizations, 23
Hearing disturbances, 124–125
Heart attack:
  emergency treatment for, 228, 230, 235–
    238, 242–243
  home-care after, 69–70
  and sex, 215–216
  signs of, 70
Heart surgery, 154–156
  and sex, 214–216
  valve, 160–161
Heat therapies, 38–39
Heimlich Maneuver, 123, 228, 232, 239–242
Hemiplegic wheelchair, 71
Hemorrhoidectomy, 161
Hemorrhoids, 235
Hernia, hiatus, 161
High-fiber diet, 142
High-protein milkshake, 145
Hints, care-giving, 25–30
Hip fracture, 301

Home attendants, 9
Home care:
  benefits, 3
  costs, 2–3, 21–25
  defined, 2
Home-Care Plan, 25–26
Home-chore services, 288
Home-health aides, 9, 14
Home-Health Chart, 16–17, 18–19
Home-study programs, 200–201
Hospice, 314–316
Hospital(s):
  ambulances, 231
  children in, 183–186
  costs, 2, 3
  discharge planning, 7
  emergency rooms, 232–233
  in-hospital hospice, 315–316
  for mentally ill, 250–251
Hospital-coordinated home care program, 7
Hostile behavior, 266–267
Housekeepers, 9
Hugging, 205–206, 222
Humidifiers, 34
Hydrocollator packs, 38
Hygiene, 40, 48–60
Hypertension, 92, 142
Hyperventilating, 98
Hypoglycemic reaction, 242
Hypotension, 92
Hysterectomy, 161–162
  and sex, 214

Ileostomy, 163, 218, 220
Immunization, 167
Impotence, 212, 218, 219, 221, 222, 224–225
Incision, surgical, 150, 152–153, 155, 159
Inclinator Company of America, 76
Incontinence, 57–58, 121–122
Independence, patient, 51, 55
Infant care:
  chronical illnesses, 190–192
  common illnesses, 167–178
  movement of infant, 44
  See also Child care
Infections:
  ear, 170–171
  urinary tract, 56, 59
Information sources, 318–329
Infra-red heat, 38

In-hospital hospice, 315–316
Injured patient, movement of, 47
Insomnia, 35–36, 104–105
Insulin, 140, 242–243
Insurance, *See* Health inusrance
Intermediate care facilities (ICF), 278–279
Internal bleeding 234–235
Intestinal disorders, 105–106
  diet for, 137–138, 144
  See also specific conditions
Intravenous feedings, 144
Itching, 108, 149

Jaundice, 106
J.T. Posey Company, 76

Kagle Home-Health Services, 75
Karaya, 164
Kidney disorders:
  and breath odor, 115
  and urine ordor, 116
Kübler-Ross, Elisabeth, 310, 313
Kussmaul respiration, 100

Lactose-restricted diet, 142
Levadopa, 208, 306
Licensed practical nurses, 12
Licensed vocational nurses, 12
Lighting, sickroom, 18
Linens, bed, 21
Liquids(s), 135–136
  diet, 138
  medication, 61
  recipes for, 144–146
  for sick children, 178–179
Listening, health clues detected by, 119–121
Lithium, 268
Low-fat/low-cholesterol diet, 139
Low-sodium diet, 142–143
Lumps, 117

Maddak Inc., 75
Major medical insurance, 22
Manic depression, 250, 267–268
MAO inhibitors, 68, 272–273
Marginal income programs, 24
Marriage, effects of child care on, 197–198
Massage, 37, 205
Mastectomy, 162–163
  and sex, 216–217

Mattress, 17–18
  protection, 21
Measles, 173–175
Meat/fish/poultry/beans food group, 127, 134
Mechanically soft diet, 137
Medicaid, 24
Medic Alert Emblem, 228
Medicare, 22, 23–24, 309
Medication:
  administering, 60–68
  child, 62, 167–168, 173, 176, 177, 196–197
  drug interaction, 68, 272–273
  elderly, 297, 306–307
  knowing about, 60
  for mentally ill, 257, 266, 268, 271–273
  and nausea, 64, 66, 133
  organization, 67
  refusal, 62–63
  and sex, 207–208
  skipped doses, 62
  types, 60, 61
  See also specific drugs
Medication Sheet, 17, 18–19, 67
Memory loss, 106
  elderly, 277, 296–298
Menstruation, 194
Mental changes in patient, 106–107
Mental illness, 249–274
  care tips for specific conditions, 263–271
  diagnosis, 253–254
  emotional repercussions to care giver, 249, 259–263
  family support groups for, 258–260, 261
  home care problems, 255–260
  hospital care, 250–251
  medication, 257, 266, 268, 271–273
  professionals, 251–254, 258–260, 274
Metropolitan Jewish Geriatric Center, NY, 32
Milk/cheese food group, 128, 134, 142, 145–146
Milkshakes, 145–146
Mineral oil, 68
Modified scooter, 72
Moisture, 117
Moles, 108
Mouth problems, 110
  diet for, 133–134
  dryness, 134
Movement of patient, 42–47

Multigeneration communes, 289
Multipurpose day care programs, 286–287
Mumps, 175
Muscular rigidity, 118
Music, 77–78

National Center for Health Services Research, 287
National Easter Seal Society, 75
National HomeCaring Council, 14
National Self-Help Clearinghouse, 195
Nausea:
  child, 178
  and diet, 133
  and medication, 64, 66, 133
  and radiation therapy, 64
Neurologists, 251
Neurotics Anonymous, 274
New York University Medical Center, 32
Nitroglycerine, 244
Nocturnal penile tumescence test, 219, 224
Noncommunicative physician, 29–30
Nose abnormalities, 107
Nosebleeds, 234
Numbness, cast, 54, 55
Nurse(s):
  choice, 12–13
  gender, 13
  licensed practical, 12
  licensed vocational, 12
  psychiatric, 251
  registered, 12
  visiting, 9, 13, 288
Nursing home(s), 272–282
  phobia, 280–281
  selection, 279–282
  types, 278–279
Nutritional therapists. *See* Dieticians

Occupational therapists, 9, 15, 294, 303–304, 305
Odors, 114–116, 220
  cast, 54
  sickroom, 34
On Death and Dying (Kübler-Ross), 310, 313
Open heart surgery, and sex, 214–215
Oral bleeding, 234
Oral contraceptives, 215, 219
Oral hygiene, 48–49
Oral problems, 110, 133–134

Oral temperature, 82–84
Orgasm, 212, 216, 221
Osteoarthritis, 293–294
Ostomy, 163–164
  and sex, 217–220

Pain, post-surgical, 151–152, 153
Painful breathing, 100
Pallor, 108–109
Pap smears, 226
Paraffin bath, 38–39
Paralysis, 221, 222, 302–303
Paramedics, 230–231
Parenteral nutrition, 144
Parkinson's disease, 208, 250, 304–307
Passive exercises, 42
Patient(s), 9–10
  administering medication, 60–68
  bathing, 48–53
  child as, 166–201
  clothing, 34–35
  complaints, 121–125
  diet, 126–147
  dignity, 27, 58
  elderly, 47, 275–308
  emergency treatment, 227–248
  entertainment, 76–79
  health clues, 95–125
  hygiene, 40, 48–60
  mentally ill, 249–274
  movement, 40, 42–47
  post-surgical, 47, 148–165
  rest and exercise tips, 35–38
  terminally ill, 309–317
  toileting, 55–60
Patient-coordinated home care program, 8–9
Penile implants, 219, 224–225
Pets, 78–79
Phlegm, 115
Phobia, nursing home, 280–281
Physical therapists, 9, 14, 303–304
Physician(s), 10, 25, 283, 316
  choice of, 11
  noncommunicative, 29–30
Physician-coordinated home care program, 7–8
Physician's Desk Reference (PDR), 60, 207
Pill Organizer, 67
Pillows, 21
Pilonidal cyst, 165
Planned Parenthood Center, 226

Plants in sickroom, 34
Post-surgical patient(s), 148–165
  movement, 47
Powdered medication, 61
Power, loss of, 122
Pregnancy, 215, 226
  and ostomy, 219
Pressure sores, 17–18, 39–42, 112
Primary care physician, 11
Private ambulances, 231
Private foundations, 24–25
Prostate surgery, and sex, 220–221
Protective services, 289
Protein, 127, 128, 132, 134, 145
Prostheses, penile, 224–225
Psychiatric nurses, 251
Psychiatrists, 251–252
Psychoanalysts, 252
Psychologists, 252
Psychotics, 250
Puberty, and chronic illness, 194–195
Pulse, 87–89, 118
Purulent discharge, 101

Quadraplegics, 223

Radial pulse, 87
Radiation therapy, 63–64, 134, 135
  child, 187–188
  diet, 139–140
Rails, bed, 21
Range of Motion exercises, 38, 42
Rashes, 109
Reagan, Ronald, 2, 309
Recipes, 144–147
Recliner wheelchair, 71
Rectal bleeding, 235
Rectal temperature, 84–86
Registered dieticians, 9, 14–15, 136
Registered nurses, 12
Reproductive health care, 226
Respiration rate, 89–90
Respiratory disorders, 98–100
Respiratory therapists, 9, 15
Rest, 35–36
Restlessness, 97
Restricted diet, 136–143
Reye's syndrome, 167–168
Rheumatoid arthritis, 293, 294–295

St. Louis Ostomy & Medical Supply, Inc., 76
Scarlet fever, 166, 175–176
Scars, post-surgical, 150, 155
Schizophrenia, 250, 269–271
Seizures, emergency treatment for, 245
Self-help aids, 74–76
Self-help groups, 8–9, 195
Semiconsciousness, 107
Senility, 63, 250, 285, 296–301
Sensation, loss of, 122–123
Sense of humor, 28
Serous discharge, 101
Sex and sexuality, 202–226
   and chronically ill adolescent, 194–195
   and depression, 205, 212, 221–222
   emotional changes, 203, 205–225
   extramarital, 215–216
   impotence, 212, 218, 219, 221, 222, 224–225
   and medication, 207–208
   post-surgical, 156, 164, 213–221
   professional help, 202, 208–211, 213, 223, 224, 225
   and specific illnesses, 211–225
Sex therapists, 202, 208–211, 213, 223, 224, 225
Sexual myopia, 204–205
Shaking, 97
Shampoos, bed, 52–53
Sheltered housing, 289–290
Shivering, 102
Shock, 117
   anaphylactic, 124, 246–247
   emergency treatment, 246–247
Shortness of breath, 98
Showers, 52
Sickroom:
   choice, 17
   cleaning, 33–34
   supplies, 17–21
Skilled nursing facilities (SNF), 278–279
Skin:
   bedsores, 17–18, 39–42, 112
   and casts, 53–55
   changes, 107–109
   dry, 48, 49
   grafts, 165
   texture, 119
Sleep, 35–36
Sleep apnea, 99–100

Snoring, 99
Social health maintenance organization, 32
Social workers, 9, 12, 195, 286
Sodium, diet low in, 142–143
Soft-solid diet, 137
Sola Designs, Inc., 75
Sores, pressure, 17–18, 39–42, 112
Sore throat, 166, 176, 177–178
Spasticity, 97
Speech, 120
Speech therapists, 9, 14
Sperm production, and chemotherapy, 66
Sphygmomanometer, 92, 93
Spinal injuries, and sex, 222–223
Sponge bath, 52
Sputum odor, 115
Stains, 34
Standard wheelchair, 71
Stereotypes, old-age, 276
Steroids, 68
Stoma, 163–164, 217–220
Stomach aches, 176–177
Stool, 55–60
   color, 110–111
   incontinence, 57–58, 121–122
   odor, 115–116
Strep throat, 166, 177–178
Stroke, 302–304
   mental problems due to, 250, 300, 303
   and sex, 221–222
Suicide, 251
Sun:
   and drugs, 68
   and incision site, 153
Supine patient, movement of, 45
Supplies, sickroom, 17–21
Suppositories, 61, 66
Surgeon, choice of, 148–149
Surgery:
   care after, 148–165
   child, 183–186
   See also types of surgery
Surgical wounds, 150, 152–153, 155, 159
Sutures, 152–153
Swallowing difficulties, 123–124
Sweating, 111
Sweets, 131, 132
Swelling, 112
   and cast, 54
Swimmer's ear, 170

Tablet medication, 61
Tantrums, child, 181–182
Tardive dyskinesia, 273
Tasks, home-care, 33–79
Taste perception, changes in, 135
Team, home-care, 9
Telephone numbers, emergency, 228, 232
Telephone reassurance programs, 290
Temperature reading, 80–87
  axillary, 86
  below normal, 104
  oral, 82–84
  rectal, 84–86
Tenderness, 118–119
Terminal illness, 309–317
  and hospice, 314–316
Tetracycline, 68
Texture, skin, 119
Therapies:
  cold, 38–39
  heat, 38–39
Therapists, 9, 14–15. *See also types of
    therapists*
Throat:
  changes, 110
  sore, 166, 176, 177–178
Time-release capsules, 61
Toileting, 55–60
Tonsillectomy, 165
Tooth brushing, 48–49
Toothette, 49
Touch, 36–37
  health clues detected by, 117–119
  and sexuality, 205–206, 222
Treatment, emergency, 227–248
Tremors, 97
Tricyclic antidepressants, 273
Troches, 61
Tub bath, 51–52
Tube feedings, 143–144
Tumors, 158–159

Ulcer diet, 137–138
Ultrasound, 39
Unconsciousness, emergency treatment for,
  247
United States Pharmacopedia/Dispensing

Information (USP/DI), 60, 207
Upjohn Healthcare Services, 13
Urinal, 56
Urinary tract infections, 56, 59
Unrine, 55–60
  color, 112–113
  incontinence, 57–58, 121–122
  odor, 116, 120
Urocare Products, Inc., 76
Urologists, 208, 226
Urostomy, 163, 218, 220

Vaginal bleeding, 235
Vaporizers, 34
Vascular surgery, 224
Vegetable/fruit food group, 127–128, 134, 142
Vegetarians, 132
Veterans services, 24
Vibrations, body, 119
Vibrators, 206
Visiting Nurse Association, 13
Visiting nurses, 9, 13, 288
Vital signs, 80–94
Vitamins, 68, 129
  A, 127–128, 129
  B, 128
  C, 127, 129, 153
Volunteers, 9, 291
Vomitus odor, 116

Walking, manner of, 96
Water:
  and drug interaction, 68
  Salt in, 143
Weight loss, 113–114, 130–132
  child, 179–180, 198, 199
  elderly, 292–293
Wet bed bath, 49
Wheelchair patients, 40, 51, 71–73
  movement of, 73
Wheelchairs, 71–73
Wheezing, 99
Whirlpool, 39
Whitaker Company, 75
Wounds, surgical, 150, 152–153, 155, 159

X-rays, 186

Mara Covell was formerly on the editorial staffs of *Vogue* and *Self* magazines. She is currently Senior Editor at the 13-30 Corporation, publisher of numerous health-related magazines in Knoxville, Tennessee.

Maurice Beer, M.D., is an internist affiliated with Beekman Downtown and Doctors hospitals in New York City.

Eileen Hanley, R.N., was director of nursing at the Manhattan Health Center in New York City and now does intensive-care nursing at New York University Hospital.